SEX EDUCATION

SEX EDUCATION

Political Issues in Britain and Europe

Philip Meredith

ROUTLEDGE
London and New York

First published 1989
by Routledge
11 New Fetter Lane, London EC4P 4EE
29 West 35th Street, New York, NY 10001

© 1989 International Planned Parenthood Federation

Printed and bound in Great Britain by
Mackays of Chatham PLC, Kent

British Library Cataloguing in Publication Data

Meredith, Philip, *1950–*
    Sex education: Political issues in Britain and Europe
    1. Europe. Schools. Sex education
    I. Title
    613.9'507104

    ISBN 0-415-00604-X

Library of Congress Cataloging in Publication Data

Meredith, Philip, 1950–
    Sex education.

    Bibliography: p.
    Includes index.
    1. Sex instruction — Great Britain. 2. Sex
instruction — Europe — Case studies. 3. Sex instruction —
Government policy — Great Britain. 4. Sex instruction —
Government policy — Europe — Case studies. I. Title.
HQ57.6.G7M47   1989   306.7'07   88-35679

    ISBN 0-415-00604-X

For I.J.M

CONTENTS

Preface

The arguments in this book have developed from a project proposal I presented to volunteers representing autonomous national Family Planning Associations (FPAs), in their capacity as members of the Europe Region of the International Planned Parenthood Federation (IPPF) in 1985. The objective of the project (see Appendix) was to further understanding of the problems surrounding the introduction of 'sex education'(1) in schools, which are common to countries with different historical, political and socio-cultural traditions. Part of this objective was to review critically the role of the FPA within the broader political management of the educational system in which sex education is located.(2) An earlier study of national provision for 'planned parenthood', had revealed that school (and therefore 'state') provision for sex education lagged significantly behind legal recognition of this subject as a component of health education.

Although few FPAs have a direct relationship with their educational systems as such, nevertheless, they are obliged, on the one hand, to find ways of helping to improve young persons' knowledge of their rights and responsibilities in this sphere. On the other, as nationally-representative interest groups, their task is to assist governments in providing the means for school teachers to operate confidently and effectively. It is argued here that to achieve this, it is necessary to understand the political dimension of their own educational strategic planning which is necessary to help the teachers negotiate the plurality of opinion on content and conduct of this subject, and the complex organisational obstacles which serve to impede as well as facilitate the educational process. The charitable status of FPAs precludes their becoming directly involved in political activities around the issues which concern them and this is not to suggest that they should. However they are obliged to plan their work with full cognisance of the political realities which so heavily dominate this subject and determine its fate.

Confronting common social problems which stem from urbanisation and the commercialisation of sexuality, most European countries are slowly moving towards the establishment of standardised curricula for school education in sexuality and personal relationships. Two interconnected problems remain which to a greater or lesser extent impede the effective integration of this subject into the broader curriculum: the first relates to the ongoing controversy over the kind of morality which such education should convey and who should be responsible for it; and secondly, what means are required to ensure sufficient teacher motivation for this subject to take its place among the 'priority' subjects which make up the curriculum. At the very least, the answer to the second problem lies in ways of reducing the disruptive effect of the first. Few European countries appear to have discovered politico-administrative structures which resolve or minimise ideological controversies such that a degree of standardisation in content and method has been achieved.

Using a similar methodology, which involved the examination of published material and interviews, eight volunteers, representing seven countries, investigated, during 1986-88, common elements in the administrative, bureaucratic or political structures through which sex education curricula are designed, as well as the more familiar moral or ideological impediments which transcend national boundaries. The report of the project is intended to furnish the IPPF with illustrations of the ways in which school-based sex education has been managed nationally (for good or bad) in respect of the organisation and regulations which are erected to control the subject, for the benefit of countries only beginning to consider state provision in this field.

This book has grown out of a contribution to the British component of this comparative work, though it is neither the work of, nor does it presume to represent the position of, the UKFPA. Rather, as a contribution to the general aims of IPPF's member associations, it does address the 'uniquely' British 'problem' of school sex education against a background of European examples researched by FPA volunteers as part of the IPPF project. As it argues in general for the inclusion of the subject in all school curricula, in particular it is a call for its inclusion as a core component of the 'National Curriculum' which the present government is in the process of creating for England and Wales. Comparative details of political management and curriculum design relating to the subject are drawn from: Sweden, Denmark, Federal Republic of Germany, Poland and Belgium, though these countries are not given equal weight. Rather, European evidence is presented which clarifies or provides alternatives to the British handling of the subject.

It focuses upon the broader 'political management' of the subject to illustrate the degree to which national politics dominates this otherwise humble part of a school curriculum. The perspective on 'State' sex education adopted here proposes that many problems conventionally regarded as 'ideological' in nature (about differences in values and facts) have in fact social structural causes and potential solutions.

Drawing upon examples of the more constructive management of the subject in Europe, the book also aims to recommend a possible course of action to those politicians and civil servants responsible for the subject in this country. However, this is not to imply that it is possible to discover a 'European' model for state sex education which may one day be adopted by all countries. The details of such a curriculum can only be 'home grown' to accord with unique elements of each country's historico-cultural background. However, there is evidence to suggest that all countries must deal, in one way or another, with the components of a supra-national guide to curriculum planning, which addresses issues both of content and organisational structure, necessary to manage the interests of national and local government, education authorities, pressure-groups and the professions.

This book is based on a conviction that, if they are permitted to do so, schools (ie. teachers) have a great potential to assist young people to make sense of the range of contradictory signals society offers them about sexuality, even though, as future parents, they may take on this role for their children. The issue for the immediate future is to discover the means to remove the destructive controversies special to Britain which prevent the establishment of a rational curriculum for school-based sex education, the teaching of which is acceptable to and defended by the *majority* of the population.

Notes

1. A term which refers to more accurately to 'education in sexuality and relationships', and includes what is termed in some countries 'family life education'.

2. The results of this comparative study will appear in Meredith, P *The Other Curriculum: European Strategies for School Sex Education* IPPF Europe, London 1989.

Acknowledgements

This book draws upon the ideas and studies of my colleagues in the Regional Advisory Group whose collective efforts I am responsible to edit elsewhere in the form of an IPPF Regional Project Report. Special thanks are therefore offered for their stimulating and challenging contributions to fulfilling the project's objectives: Hélène Aronis and Freddy Deven (Belgium), Alan Beattie (UK), Claus Drunkeknmölle (German Democratic Republic), Mikolaj Kozakiewicz (Poland), Karl Plümer (Federal Republic of Germany), Hanne Risør (Denmark). Meeting in different European capitals over three years, this small group was kindly awarded the financial means by the IPPF European Regional Council, to share and explore inroads into this most difficult subject, some of which had to be abandoned, others which provided a common formula for all the resulting country case studies.

I am particularly indebted to UKFPA volunteer, Alan Beattie, many of whose ideas appear and are drawn upon in this study.

This work has also relied upon the assistance given by individuals who played leading roles in the establishment of state school sex education in their countries. Thanks are extended in particular to Carl Gustav Boëthius, Secretary to the Swedish National Board of Education Commission on sex education which sat in the 1970s and created the guidelines for school practice in operation throughout Sweden today; and to his Danish equivalent, Chairman of the 1960s Danish National Commission on school state education, the late Ingolf Leth.

I am indebted to the willingness of politicians, FPA staff, sex educators, medical and teaching professionals, inspectors of schools, civil servants and others, in seven countries who offered their time for interviews, and who must remain anonymous.

In particular, UKFPA chairperson, Dilys Cossey provided an invaluable service by conveying to me all relevant parliamentary papers. IPPF Deputy Secretary-General Donald Lubin and Assistant Secretary-General, Pramilla Senanayake have continued to be supportive of this extra-project initiative since it was proposed in 1987. I would also like to extend apologies and thanks to my colleagues in the Programme Department of the IPPF for their tolerance of regular absences during the time this manuscript was being completed. Thanks also to Jim Dewar, John Fell and Fiona Heald for guiding the manuscript to the publisher.

Although written on behalf of the IPPF, as a staff member, I am not representing here the views of any participants in the project, the Europe Region or the Federation, but am alone responsible for the content of and any weaknesses in arguments presented.

PART 1 : SCHOOL SEX EDUCATION IN BRITAIN

Chapter 1

The Sexual Politics of the Classroom

Although a subject of continuing controversy in many developed societies, by the 1980s, sex education in one form or another has become a nominal part of the curricula of most of their schools. Whatever impediments exist to its continued refinement, which are thrown up by the historical-cultural background of these societies, the majority of European governments recognise, in principle, that they must act to equip young people with the means to understand and protect their own reproductive health and potential; and that the rapid changes taking place in societies demand that parents and the Churches be assisted in this through the formal education process.

If it is accepted that schools (teachers) do have a legitimate and productive role to play in the sexual socialisation of young people, it remains to be seen to what extent they can undertake this task efficiently, enthusiastically and in accord with the wishes of the populations they exist to serve. The problems which follow from a 'formalisation' of what has traditionally been a hidden, furtive, taboo-ridden, even unconscious area of learning for many are many and complex. In some societies the subject has been plagued by moral controversy and even scandal; Britain has suffered exceptionally in this respect, though it is not unique.

This book aims to clarify the problem of establishing sex education as an uncontroversial component of the school curriculum. It is based on a conviction that the logic behind the introduction of this subject into a state education system leads necessarily towards standardisation of the content and mode of teaching, and that the best way to achieve this lies in a 're-construction' of the sex education curriculum in all its detail sufficient to gain a minimum of required public understanding of and support for what is being proposed.

The aim is to reveal sex education as a national political issue par excellence, and to show that where progress has been made in Europe this has taken a national political character. In the form of a component of state school education, the subject is too contentious to be delegated to a local authority or non-governmental level with any measure of success. Sooner or later, the authority brought by government is required to establish sex education practice, though the *manner* in which this is achieved is critical.

1

At present, surveys inform us that school sex education in Britain has the *tacit* acceptance of the majority of parents. However, it is likely that such support is more for the principle of, rather than particular programme of sex education practice; a support which may rapidly erode in the face of controversy, real or convoluted. It is unfortunate that this subject's recent historical evolution has been determined more by the consequences of 'moral panic' than rationalisation.

Although sex education in school raises practical political issues of human rights, participation and democracy, it is more often discussed as a matter of acceptable or unacceptable sexual ethics. Once integrated into the school system, political administration and sexual ethics become dialectically related. Solutions to divisions over the latter in practice become dependent upon how the former is organised. The aim here is to illustrate this interrelationship by comparing the development of the subject in Britain (or more strictly in organisational terms, England) with that in a selection of other European countries.

The comparative development of the subject in Europe offers valuable insights into how the subject has been managed politically in order to remove, minimise or otherwise circumvent the destructive doubts and antagonisms which drive the subject into a hidden corner of the curriculum. These are issues with which other European countries have grappled more and less successfully (or are in the process of confronting now). To a certain, though indeterminate degree, the philosophical, psychological and physical dilemmas attached to formal education in sexual relationships transcend political and socio-cultural boundaries. It is this level of commonality, and the lessons Britain may learn from the comparison, which is the subject here.

Perspectives on School Sex Education

From the scientific point of view, the outstanding problem of existing school-based sex education in developed countries lies in discovering the means to measure and then increase its effect on adolescent sexual behaviour, with the longer term aim of reducing the numbers of unplanned pregnancies or incidence of sexually-transmitted diseases. At least this is the direct return most governments expect in having the educational system cater for what was traditionally the exclusive domain of parents.

However, drawing upon the most extensive research undertaken, in the USA despite the fact that 80% of school districts offer instruction in sex related topics, the best that can be claimed for these courses, as discovered by attitude surveys, is that those adolescents who had received sex education were more able to discuss the subject with their parents. Sex education as currently taught has little if any effect on the decision of young people to initiate sexual activity or on the incidence of pre-marital pregnancy, though it may effect use of contraceptives during the sexual debut.(1) Better claims are made for the school sex education offered in Sweden, although scientific explanation of the processes at work there is as lacking as anywhere else.(2)

By contrast, from the social point of view, the problem presented by the involvement of schools in providing adolescents with education in this subject lies in the kind of moral code within which the education is set, and the degree to which parents can influence this *vis-à-vis* the formal educator. No country is immune from the apparently universal conviction among many that the power which education brings is potentially as corrupting as ennobling, and that education in sexuality will carry with it the threat of experimentation by the immature, leading to the very consequences that this education was intended to prevent. At risk of over-simplification this matter usually appears in the form of 'traditionalistic' (pro-parent, anti-school) versus 'progressive' (pro-parent, pro-school) opinion.

An objection to school-based sex education has been voiced by at least one progressive pro-sex education movement, on the grounds that no sexually-liberating education can be provided within the context of what is in practice felt by many of its clients to be a repressive institution.(3) Other critics of 'state' sex education, such as psychiatrist Thomas Szasz, base their doubts upon the willingness of government ministries of education to refrain from manipulating the subject for political ends unconnected with the subject.(4)

In spite of these caveats, it is likely that the global movement toward governmental endorsement of, and direct support for, a school-based sex education, outside of direct parental control, will continue. Anticipating the conflict which must inevitably stem from re-negotiating basic rights to educate in such a moral sphere, the United Nations recommendation 29 of the Mexico City Conference on Population in August 1984 is carefully worded to avoid offence:

> 'Governments are urged to ensure that adolescents, both boys and girls, receive adequate education, including family life and sex education, with due consideration given to the role, rights and obligations of parents, and changing individual and cultural values. Suitable family planning information and services should be made available to adolescents within the changing socio-cultural framework of each country.'(5)

In theory, there are powerful justifications for school-based sex education, even if this influence is likely always to remain less than that of the mass media and peers. Whatever its drawbacks, the classroom provides the most formalised, controllable and durable access to adolescents as a 'captive audience', over a critical period of learning and psycho-social development. Although it has been argued that young people can be reached more powerfully and persuasively through use of the media, this is always likely to be far more piecemeal, occasional and impersonal than through person-to-person learning. Moreover, the authority invested in the school as purveyor of 'factual' knowledge awards it a status in theory which stands above the parent, in addition to the random sources of information from the surrounding society. The school potentially offers the young person a source of legitimacy, a yardstick by which the values of the family and society may be judged.

This being so, to seek to shift responsibility from traditional sources of sexual-moral education to the formal institution of the school makes it incumbent upon governments (or their ministries of education) to provide the means for teachers to undertake this unique and difficult dimension of education. Evidence collected by the IPPF in 1985 on the situation regarding provision for school sex education in 19 European countries indicates that very few governments have seriously confronted the issues raised by this shift.(6) In 1985, 9 European countries had created legal provision for school sex education, with a further 2 in the process of creating such legislation (7). By contrast, not one country investigated by its national FPA, with the exception of Sweden, reported that sufficient technical provision had been forthcoming for such 'enabling' laws to have the widespread impact desired. In fact, an impasse has been created by the gesture of legal provision which has surpassed the ability of the state apparatus to address and resolve the complex problems which such provision raises, irrespective of the national culture.

Governmental authority and legitimacy have been required to undertake the process of establishing state school provision of sex education (even if in name only) in all European countries in which it has been established. The very involvement of the state school system brings with it an extensive politico-bureaucratic apparatus. It has been a high price to pay for the progress gained in this field in view of the unproductive though inevitable 'interference effect' created by the various sub-rationales and motives by direct parts of this apparatus. Hence the doubt expressed by Szasz, reflecting upon the subject in Britain and the USA:

> 'The term sex education conceals more than it reveals. It conceals the specific social, educational, and economic policies used to implement sex education, the moral values secretly encouraged and discouraged; and last but not least, the problems that derive

inexorably from involving the school system - and hence the government - in defining what constitutes education in human sexuality.'(8)

In her discussion of a familiar impediment to sex education practice in the classroom - the need to create a vocabulary to conceptualise the subject which permits communication with the 'consumer' as well as the 'provider'- Carol Lee makes passing reference to one minor part of this apparatus. This relates to the power exercised by administrative bodies, members of which operate according to unknown and unexpressable criteria and motives which have their origin in their own psycho-sexual development, but which must be negotiated by the educator.(9) It is to the operation of and relations between such bodies that one must look for the roots of the school sex education dilemma, as well as the 'superstructure' of Parliamentary and media debate of the ethical issues alone.

Sex Education in British Schools: The Political Context

The project on which this study is based began in late 1985. At that time, the structure of British school education was perceived to be the principal impediment to progress in sex education on any coordinated national scale. At that time the general secretary of the UKFPA, Alastair Service, summarised the situation thus:

'Given the control of curriculum by individual schools (rather than by government policy) in Britain, it is difficult to recommend realistic action by Government. It is understood that in liaison committees between the Department of Health and the Department of Education, the health needs of young people for education on sex and planned parenthood are frequently urged. The Department of Education has moved cautiously to encourage schools to provide this in the context of Health Education, but little has been heard since the 1981 School Curriculum document was published. Schools are required since that time to notify the Department of Education about their sex education programmes, and the DHSS (Department of Health and Social Security) might best pursue the matter by asking for a progress report and then suggesting next steps.'(10)

The developments which have occurred since this time have transformed the politico-bureaucratic management of the subject beyond recognition. The creation of a plan for a national curriculum of core subjects, and the centralisation of control over the substance of these and 'fringe' subjects including sex education will have far-reaching consequences on what teachers are willing to offer under this heading. The spectre of AIDS has also led to changes in the manner in which sex education is taught. Both events potentially have both negative and positive longer term consequences for the subject.

The debate over school sex education in Britain has rarely been balanced and dispassionate, though in recent years it has become increasingly rather than less controversial. According to recent research by the Washington-based Population Crisis Committee, Britain offers perhaps the most comprehensive, free contraceptive service in the world.(11) Yet this contrasts strikingly with the exceptional difficulties it has in establishing an uncontroversial moral education within the school curriculum, despite its need being recognised by power-holders of all political persuasions, as well as the public. This phenomenon is yet to be fully explained.

Unlike in other European countries, there is no explicit government provision for the inclusion of sex education in the school curriculum as such, though there has been a stream of somewhat guarded and often ambiguous 'guidelines' aimed at schools from 'official' sources concerning what is or is not permissible/advisable to teach. The national curriculum has been created as a means of improving the standards of 'essential' (technical) subjects, and is therefore not explicitly concerned with 'values' as such. However, the present Conservative government has also chosen to become involved with the content as well as organisation of schooling; and this extends to the contentious issue of the values which schools are expected to reflect.

However, such are the philosophical divisions in British society, exacerbated by shifts in public attitudes to socialistic and conservative thinking, that such potentially positive developments for the organisational efficiency of education are likely to suffer from this wider political climate. For more complex, though not unconnected, reasons, sex education has been expressedly omitted from the plans for a national curriculum at this time. No national authority exists at present with the necessary mandate to establish guidelines on the content and direction of the subject sufficient for its inclusion, however tangentially. This is unfortunate as such inclusion is the only long term means of resolving the fundamental dilemmas which it raises. There is an unfortunate circularity in the argument which must conclude that until it becomes an accepted part of a national curriculum, it will remain a subject of arbitrary content, hidden curriculum and attendant controversy, though this is the one reason for its inadmissability.

Current Provision in Schools

From the point of view of our sociological knowledge, the classroom setting remains an almost totally hidden realm in respect of sex education. So sensitive is the subject, from the highest to most parochial political level, there is great reluctance to permit observation of the teaching process. To date, it has been necessary to rely upon descriptive measures of 'quantity' rather than 'quality'. Indeed this is how many pro-sex education campaigners and researchers continue to address the shortcomings of the subject - by demanding that 'more' should be given. It is necessary to move beyond this reaction to identify and understand impediments to practice. Over the last 25 years, surveys such as those by Schofield, Farrell, and Kozakiewicz and Rea, have identified shortcomings. (12) Moral conservatives compete with liberals in defining what sex education approach is required to reflect their respective images of a good society. The few 'qualitative' accounts (13) are even more critical than quantitative studies.

The most important recent research undertaken on the subject in British schools is by Isobel Allen (14). This attempts to offer an estimate of quality and quantity in an effort to forestall recent political measures to introduce rights of parental withdrawal of children from such classes. She questioned pupils and their parents in a geographical spread of around 200 families, with the objective of identifying 'to what extent present (sex education) provision was meeting needs' with the condition that 'it was important to establish exactly what was being taught at school'. It was discovered that there has been 'an enormous increase' in the provision of education in sex and personal relationships in British secondary schools, and that the subject has become more integrated into the whole school curriculum. The research confirmed that 95% of teenage pupils and 96% of parents believed that schools should (continue to) provide sex education (27% of parents believing that it should be the *sole* responsibility of schools).

What is so startling about this exhaustive survey is the difference between the general picture it paints of relatively widespread provision and satisfied clients, compared with the darker picture painted by the critics in the media. One could argue that it is the latter medium which has had the greater impact on political decision-making concerning the management of the subject. Is sex education really being taught to the satisfaction of the spectrum of interests in the society or not? Allen's findings present a picture which is influenced by the methodology used and the target groups approached (questionnaires aimed to elicit the opinions of pupils and parents, though not teachers). While it is an important addition to our knowledge of the subject that those questioned believed that teenagers gained most information they had about sexuality from schools, it is not comforting to read that 43% of parents surveyed were 'satisfied' with the sex education the schools provided, without knowing how much these parents actually knew about this teaching, or about those who were not so satisfied. The conclusion drawn by Allen is a central finding of the research, though nevertheless fails to pursue its significance for the future development of the subject in schools:

> 'It should be stated immediately that the wish by parents for secondary schools to provide their children with the facts about reproduction, puberty, pregnancy and childbirth, contraception, abortion, venereal disease, homosexuality and so on, was reinforced by the wish for the schools to provide their children with education on such matters as family and parenthood, personal relationships, feelings and emotions and understanding the opposite sex'(15)...'there was a great desire among parents that teenagers should receive "proper" education on these topics...'(16)

Again one is left with the feeling that a single reality is being observed from two perspectives which fail to connect: that portrayed by the survey, and the political reality which exists in the public consciousness, courtesy of the mass media - concerned with the moral interpretation of 'facts'. What fails to be addressed in the reported comments of parents and the interpretation of the researcher is the fundamental question: what are teachers to present to young people as the 'facts' about, for example, 'contraception' or 'homosexuality', and how did they come by such facts and the educational meaning derived from them?

In its original common use and sense, 'sex education', on which all sexual reform movements have based their case, referred to the transmission of factual knowledge to the young in appropriate ways in order to release them from problems arising from ignorance of their bodies and the nature of relationships. The assumption here was that the potential unhappiness which so often stems from sexual life may be minimised through knowledge. In this albeit naïve sense, sex education has conventionally been seen as a way of achieving sensual satisfaction without sexual pathology or unwanted pregnancy. This is still the meaning implied by most who complain of insufficient provision of such education, assuming the problem to be one of insufficient knowledge. However, the 'factual' basis of sexuality as understood here, viz: a collection of scientifically-grounded descriptions and explanations of constant socio-biological phenomena *to which* desired values may be attached is no longer tenable.(See chapter 3).

The central problem for sex education is the identification of appropriate sources of authority required to provide a legitimacy for 'factual' presentations of sexuality and their social meaning. Parents may be excused in thinking the school is in a position to decide what is 'proper', though the (national) political conflicts which dominate the management of this subject in the 1980s suggest that the school alone can no longer supply the necessary legitimacy for the approach taken by its teachers. It is worth recalling that as far back as 1975, a survey by Kozakiewicz and Rea concluded that, in Britain, teachers felt that sex education was the most difficult subject to teach and the subject they were least trained to handle (17). The situation has become far more complicated since even that time. For example, a 'substantial minority' of parents interviewed by Allen believed that the school should not give moral guidance on sexual matters - simply 'education'. In its final analysis, Allen's study argues that what is problematic is more the 'delivery' than 'content' of sex education; a problem which can be resolved by the training of school teachers and persons from bona fide organisations such as marriage guidance counsellors, family planning workers, health visitors:

> 'the discriminating use of outsiders giving talks or leading discussions at schools should be encouraged' and, 'Priority should be given to training teachers in the skills needed to handle these topics in the classroom.'(18)

In the past it was sufficient that the bona fide professions which included school teachers be left collectively to iron out the extremes or biases which might be introduced by individual practitioners. In a climate in which little in sex education is not held up for scrutiny by self-appointed members of the clergy, press or Parliament, the notion of 'expertise' in this field, acquired on the basis of professional interest alone, is no longer self-evident but must be defended.

Of the 'front line' of sex education - the classroom - very little is still known, because of its inaccessibility to any kind of qualitative sociological research, especially concerning such a sensitive subject. In the present climate one can hardly blame teachers for wishing to keep it this way, as few subjects can be so professionally unrecognised, and at the same time fraught with risks to a teachers' professional integrity, under the weight of 'public concern' for 'correct' teaching. Within the new core curriculum, there are to be established measures of teacher proficiency in virtually every subject *but* health or sex education. Insofar as this area is not subject to assessment, 'specialisation' in it is hardly a rational approach to career development, even if there existed a single set of guidelines covering the theory and practice of sex education in the school curriculum. This sad state of affairs is reflected even in the absence of a common stand by the teaching profession itself. On 29th May 1987, the *Independent* newspaper reported that:

> 'Head teachers in the UK narrowly avoided a damaging split yesterday over sex education. At the annual conference of the National Association of Head Teachers there was a heated debate over whether lessons on homosexuality should be included in the

school curriculum. However, delegates finally voted to back the traditional stance on morality taken in the existing Education Act.'

There are powerful disincentives for government as well as teachers to become too involved with the problems of British school sex education (unless forced into action by scandal). For, unlike in mathematics or biology, there exists no sufficient consensus on what teachers should be empowered to teach in such a highly value-laden area. Moreover, the subject is unlikely to win votes for any political party in power in view of the antagonistic (moral) interest groups which it attracts.

Virtually everyone supports the 'principle' of sex education in schools, few agree on the details. For everyone is equally particular about what *they* define as good sex education and what they believe is permissible for children and young people to learn in school. There is little substantial debate on the subject of sex education partly because there is no clear agenda for such a debate. For some, sex education is the transmission of whatever information and guidance is necessary to combat ignorance on matters of hygiene, reproduction and sexual rights, which otherwise lead to undesirable consequences such as sexually-transmitted disease, unwanted pregnancy, sexual violence or abuse. For others, 'sex education' refers to moral instruction which is designed to withhold information until the school period is completed, or to delay awareness and choice until as late in adolescence as possible.

The situation suggests that certain basic conditions must be fulfilled if any progress is to be made nationally in ensuring that all school pupils benefit from a standardised, rational and well-taught curriculum in the future. This demands that at least some of the major antagonisms between interest groups be resolved.

Conclusion: The Lessons from Europe

In Britain, it is difficult to perceive any signs of a consensus among different groups of decision-makers over what should be taught in the classroom, nor how parental rights to socialise their children can be integrated with the right and obligation of the state to ensure that young people receive adequate health and sex education to become responsible citizens.

A nationally coordinated strategic plan for the development of the subject would need to address three issues: firstly, the respective roles, obligations, rights and responsibilities of parents and the state (ie. teachers in state schools) must be specified in detail and regulated. Secondly, it is necessary to standardise the content and delivery of such education in a way which antagonistic interest groups will not seek to undermine. Thirdly, details must be negotiated to gain the support of a maximum number of interest groups for a universal programme to be a future possibility.

In a democratic society, minority dissenters are obliged to concede the wishes of the majority. This must in principle apply to the details of sex education as much as those subjects proposed for the core curriculum in Britain. The qualitative difference between biology and sex education can only be minimised if an explicit pedagogic formula is devised for the separation and respective teaching of facts and values suitable to the pluralistic nature of contemporary British society.

Education must aim to increase social cohesion while accommodating social pluralism. The alternative is to authorise a system which imposes the values of a minority. Neither a broadly traditionalistic nor liberal sex education programme is desirable if few teachers are likely to undertake to teach it due to personal resistance or external pressure. Such a curriculum must have a practical chance of being accepted by the majority.

There are elements of this dilemma which are common to all European societies, Catholic, Christian, post-Christian and Marxist. All societies which have had their school systems address the subject of sexual socialisation have found it necessary to deal with the struggle between 'traditionalistic' and 'progressive' sentiments. All such countries have found it necessary to resort to national (or Federal) government to adjudicate in the clarification and standardisation of the teaching of sex education. More specifically, other European countries have their own more or less turbulent histories of discovering the political and scientific mechanisms for establishing state school sex education. Some have been able to apply their political systems to the task more successfully than others in removing controversy from the subject while accommodating the above interests. Nevertheless, comparative research discussed in this study reveals that a commonality of direction appears in all.

It is proposed here that Britain may have something to learn from European experiences. Although still grappling with the basic task of creating a public agenda for discussion of sexual socialisation as a component of public education, the present government has embarked upon a standardisation of the core school curriculum. This seems to remove obstacles to consensus on some curriculum issues which can be created by local educational autonomy.

The present government has taken steps to reform education in general (in the form of a national curriculum) and intervened in sex education in particular (in respect of albeit crude guidelines on national 'fundamental values'). Whatever the purpose this administration had in changing the system, the possibility has been created for the longer term resolution of problems of sex education teaching which have precedents in Europe.

As most developed societies are characterised by social pluralism, social cohesion may be maintained through a system of local autonomy or clarification of fundamental social values from the centre. In practice, modern societies most effectively operate by means of a working combination of both. In terms of British school sex education, local autonomy operates in the form of powers granted to school managers, now assisted by centrally devised 'guidelines'. It remains to be seen how efficiently the new system will operate.

The idea of a cross-national European comparison of the political management of school sex education is not based on any assumption that this uniquely British version of the problem might be resolved by adoption of a system devised in Europe, nor even that the problem has been 'solved' there. However, this does not logically exclude the possibility that techniques of ordering and conveying this knowledge used elsewhere cannot be drawn upon and developed within another social and political context .

Notes

1. editorial: 'Sex education and sex-related behaviour' in *Family Planning Perspectives* Vol 18 Number 4 July/August 1986.

2. Boëthius, C G *Current Sweden* No 315 Svenska Institutet, Box 7434 S-103 91 Stockholm 1984.

3. see chapter 6.3 regarding the position of *Pro Familia*, the FPA of the Federal Republic of Germany during the 1970s.

4. Szasz, T 'The Case against Sex Education' *British Journal of Medicine* Vol 8 December 1981.

5. United Nations: *Report of the International Conference on Population* Mexico City 6-14 August 1984 UN New York 1984 (E/conf 76/19).

6. Meredith, P and Thomas, L eds. *Planned Parenthood in Europe* Croom Helm, London 1986 pg 132.

7. Austria, Denmark, Finland, France, German Democratic Republic, Hungary, Norway, Sweden, Yugoslavia. Legislation is imminent in the Netherlands and Portugal.

8. Szasz,T op cit. pg 6.

9. Lee, Carol *The Ostrich Position* Readers and Writers, London 1983 pgs 2-4.

10. Meredith and Thomas op cit. pg 236.

11. Population Crisis Committee *World Access to Birth Control* Washington DC 1987.

12. Schofield, M *The Sexual Behaviour of Young People* Longman London 1965; *The Sexual Behaviour of Young Adults* Allen Lane, London 1973; Farrell, C *My Mother Said ...The Way Young People Learned about Sex* Routledge & Kegan Paul 1978; Kozakiewicz, M and Rea, N *Sex Education and Adolescence in Europe* IPPF Europe London 1975.

13. Lee, Carol 1983 ibid.

14. Allen, Isobel *Education in Sex and Personal Relationships* Policy Studies Institute 1987.

15. ibid. pg 178.

16. ibid pg 180.

17. Kozakiewicz, M and Rea, N 1975 op cit. pg 38 ff.

18. Allen, I 1987 op cit. pg 205. It is unfortunate that this study passed over one of its more important findings: that parents were less likely to mention the moral component of sex education, 'though they were more likely than their children to say that teachers should give guidance or help on how to behave in sexual matters' (pg 184). Most parents will indeed be trusting of teachers, until critics present information to change their minds. In the absence of rules governing method and content, parental support of individual teachers under fire is likely to be as fickle as it is vague.

Chapter 2

The Perception of School Sex Education in Parliament

Controversies surrounding school sex education have continued unabated in spite of the fact that the last 20 years have seen a great deal of applied research and curriculum options created for use by teachers in the classroom. During the 1960s and 1970s, the educational system encouraged such research and welcomed the contributions of independent organisations and individuals to 'progressive' teaching programmes, chosen from an ever increasing range of commercially-produced teaching aids.

Unfortunately, these efforts have done little to assure certain politicians and sections of the public that what teachers provide in the classroom by way of sex education is something in which they can have confidence. Indeed, selected 'progressive' sex education programmes have been held up as examples of a decline in moral standards, a free-for-all among teachers in educating pupils according to their own preferred sexual code. The extent to which such scare-mongering by a relatively small lobby has created antipathy to what are seen as certain elements within the teaching profession is reflected in the changes which the present government has felt necessary to make, particularly reflected in guidelines for teaching moral values, and reminders to teachers of their obligations to the law.

The purpose of this chapter is to identify the most important elements in the controversy over school sex education teaching. The relative obsession of the newspaper media with this subject must have played a part in ordering public consciousness of this subject. However, it is the effect of this construction of 'reality' on those power-holders who are in a position to make real changes in the educational system which concerns us here. An invaluable insight into the differing perspectives and strength of feelings which surround this subject may be gained from the Parliamentary debates in which it is raised. As Davies has noted, the attitudes and moral outlook of Members of Parliament are particularly important because they are the people who have had the power to determine the legal framework within which ordinary citizens' sexual behaviour takes place. Furthermore, insofar as the law has an effect on the moral thinking of those subject to it, the shift in moral outlook of Members of Parliament in turn affects the moral outlook of the members of the public.(1)

14

In taking this approach, it would be wrong to give the impression that Parliament has systematically addressed the problems which beset this issue in a serious way. Sex education has rarely been debated in either the House of Commons or Lords. However, on those occasions when it has been the subject of debate, it is possible to see clearly why so little progress has been made in reaching that minimum 'political consensus' which would be necessary for the subject to be organised nationally with the confidence of most major interests taken into account as has been achieved elsewhere in Europe.

This chapter draws extensively upon speeches made in both Houses during 1976 and 1986, to which is attached a commentary which aims to draw out what are believed to be the most important issues facing the subject today. However counter-productively at times, the Parliamentary debates presented below do ultimately expose the theoretical and practical issues which lie behind the easily-made pleas for better school sex education. A clear evolution takes place between the 1976 and 1986 perception of these issues.

At their worst, these speeches display the manifest ignorance, fantasies and prejudices, on both sides of the political spectrum, which have so often appeared in the press. However, they also reveal genuine anxieties over fundamental weaknesses in the organisation and management of sex education, as well as signs of more sensible attempts to grapple with the subject in a constructive way. The two debates focus upon two inter-related though easily confused approaches to the subject: firstly, the means by which a suitable moral-ideological basis for state school education in sexuality and personal relationships can be established. This refers to the necessary (and unnecessary) components of the 'knowledge base' from sexology suitable to the school context. Secondly, there are interspersed discussions of the appropriate social or organisational structure required to govern the delivery of the subject which ensures the positive commitment of all concerned.

1976 and 1986: The 'Progressive and Traditionalist Lobbies'

In recent times, 10 years elapsed between two debates which directly or indirectly came to focus on the issue. In 1976, a lengthy debate in the House of Lords tackled the question of the rectitude of government financial support to the United Kingdom Family Planning Association for its work in, among other things, providing information and education services on sex education and family planning to health and teaching professionals (in the form of educational courses) and to the public (in the form of informational literature and other publications). This discussion provides an invaluable insight into perceptions of contemporary practice and the problems posed.

It will be noticed that in spite of the gap, the subsequent debate on sex education in British schools, within the context of the 1986 Education Bill, returns to the themes which preoccupied the Lords ten years previously. There is not only little sign of progress made in reaching common ground on which the two lobbies might establish a rational and constructive dialogue on behalf of adolescents and their parents in this second confrontation, but this debate takes places in perhaps a more antagonistic atmosphere than prevailed in 1976. Only (most of) the actors have changed.

As with other foci of difference between 'right' and 'left', there is no absolute division between the respective political parties. However, a division clearly crosses the two debates in the form of opposing tendencies to which Members of the Houses ally themselves.

One tendency gravitates to a perception of sex education as a rightful domain of the teaching profession in alliance with specialist organisations delegated to design courses. There is a conviction that this education should be somewhat progressive, dealing more bluntly and from an earlier age with the moral issues of the day. Such education should aim to free adolescents from repression and ignorance, acquainting girls in particular with knowledge of family planning and reproduction in order to increase their status, independence and long-term careers. This tendency wishes to correct the inadequacies of its adherents' own school education, believing that sex education should begin early in the school career with the objective of inculcating in the young a responsible and confident attitude to their nascent sexual lives. It is likely to accept the morality of sexual relations as a trial for a marriage relationship, and that young people are likely to experiment with sex whatever their parents might prefer. It also recognises the claims of sexual minorities to tolerance though it is generally unsure about how this issue might be broached in the classroom.

This tendency also has an implicit belief in openness, the need for moral education to be a sharing of experiences - learning as a solution to irrational behaviour. In this respect, it projects a faith in the education system and in particular a trust in teachers to teach the right thing. It believes that teachers should address sexuality more openly and positively than in the past, in order to alleviate some of the responsibility which parents must also bear in this sphere. To this extent, this group also has a general faith in progressive teaching solutions to the problem of unplanned pregnancy. For convenience, this 'ideal-type' will be referred to as the 'progressive lobby'.

This dichotomy identifies, in opposition, a tendency which might be termed 'traditionalist'. Within this lobby may be found those inside and outside Parliament who object to the notion of sex education at all, though such

16

exponents are in a small minority. A larger minority argue that the school has no place usurping the rightful role of parents. Most, however, are simply committed to a version of sex education which is traditionalistic in nature. They are not convinced that teachers are to be trusted to provide the appropriate form of education, nor are they sympathetic to any approach termed 'progressive'. At its extreme such sex education as is necessary to give outside of the home should aim to *delay* the acquisition of knowledge of sexuality and contraception for as long as possible into the adolescent period, and what is given should be taught with a 'deterrent' effect in mind. This approach is based on what might be termed an 'aversion therapy' approach to socialisation and behavioural change, grounded in the philosophy of the 'less you know the less you will be concerned' and the converse conviction that 'the more you know the more you will desire to experience'. Such adherents are not convinced of the merits of responsibility through education in this sphere, and place a far greater emphasis than is fashionable on the more traditional role of women concerning marriage, the family and childbearing.

Perhaps in earlier times when the mass media was not so all pervasive; when it did not offer sexuality as a commodity to a 'teenage' as well as adult 'market', there might have been much more public and professional sympathy for the latter conviction. However, the inexorable consequences of post-war mass culture, which influences all but the very young, have necessitated a search for alternative solutions to social problems particularly within education which has carried a large section of the public with it.

It is a central characteristic of the oppositional stalemate of the battle for British school sex education that the two lobbies gravitate to conservative and socialistic-liberal political positions from which to defend their ideological ground and attack the opposition. Particularly in recent politics, it is evident that *sex education has been deployed as a vehicle for right- versus left-wing antagonism*, although, as has been noted, it is less accurate to divide the debate along *party* political lines.

In common with many other European countries in the post-war era, sections of British society have attempted through liberal legislation to introduce a more sexually open and sexually positive society. Several laws passed in the 1960s and 1970s aimed to shift the balance of control over sexual behaviour from the state to the individual. There has nevertheless always been a substantial resistance to the drift toward sexual liberalisation, which has increased vocally and numerically with the ascendancy of Conservative party power during the 1980s. In the field of sex education, the recent changes in the education system contain elements of a moral 'counter-revolution', the future course of which cannot be guessed at this time.

The 1976 House of Lords Debate on the Role of the Family Planning Association

On 14th January 1976, the House of Lords began a major debate on the role of the Family Planning Association (FPA) and the status of this non-governmental organisation as a government-funded training and information service. The debate quickly shifted focus to an examination of school sex education per se. The two interconnected and recurrent themes of this debate concern: the values which should govern the teaching of sexuality and relationships; and, what constitutes a suitable qualification to undertake the task on a national scale.

The FPA was recognised as being in a position to play such a pivotal role in the kind of education being provided in schools for no other reason than that few other sources of expertise existed on which teachers could rely to obtain the basic knowledge and teaching method they required (this is discussed further in chapter 3). This state of affairs was a source of considerable anxiety to Baroness Elles and other conservative members considering the gravity of the subject in their eyes:

'Unlike the teaching of other subjects, such as history, geography,... which are concerned with the imparting of information and the extension of knowledge...sex education can and does influence not only the mental understanding of a child but also has, or may have, an immediate and future impact on patterns of behaviour, social attitudes, emotional, psychological and physical experience...What is sex education about? It does not deal only with sexual matters... It also deals with moral education. It can have the effect of bringing up children to live according to the rules accepted by society as being reasonable and in the best interests of all within society, or it can be directed to changing the climate and mores of society. Therefore the importance attached to this subject is considerable, equally in the manner in which it is taught, in who teaches it, in the aims and objectives of those who teach it, in where it is taught, in the effects of such teaching....'(2)

The import of the teaching of sex education to 'captive audiences' of school pupils places Baroness Elles and others in a dilemma. For the principle of conducting sex education within a broader school-based health education was gradually being accepted by both sides of the political spectrum.

However, recognition of the 'need' for an education to ensure the health and welfare of young people had preceded the creation of a curriculum to achieve this *which is more or less acceptable to most if not all shades of moral/political opinion.* As a result, head teachers and teachers have been forced to rely upon their own judgement in deciding the content and delivery of the subject, making use of what is available in the non-governmental sector. This sector comprised independent national charities such as the FPA or National Marriage Guidance Council; relatively independent government established 'advisory' organisations such as the Health Education Council, the establishment media bodies such as the BBC; and the wide range of similarly independent educational institutions, and individuals who contributed to the nascent field through research and publication. The government, itself, had turned to bona fide organisations such as the FPA and the NMGC because of their recognised pioneering work in the general field of sexuality and relationship counselling, if not school sex education as such.

The 1976 debate revealed the critical fact that Elles and other critics in the Lords refused to accept the government endorsement of these organisations or their bona fide status. On the side of 'progressive' education, the government of the day (Labour) had failed to retain the confidence of the moral right. In fact, the moral right remained highly suspicious of the above organisations, believing them, rightly or wrongly, to be allied in their philosophy and practice to what it believed to be the 'libertarian' left. On this, the right proclaimed it was speaking for a large proportion of head teachers, teachers, politicians, health professionals and parents. Neither the government nor those sympathetic to the 'progressive' movement in education chose to disclaim this openly.

More important is Elles' and her fellow Lords' distrust of the teaching profession to provide an 'acceptable' sex education, and the fact that, in the privacy of the classroom, this profession remains outside of (political) control. The debate revealed this to a be a source of great anxiety for the traditionalist tendency in the Lords, several of whose adherents speculated upon the profession's subversive potential in this area:

'We must not let loose on the children people who are not qualified... It is not the qualification which the teacher has that matters but the character of the teacher... 'Pupils are at the mercy of their teachers... the right instruction will be given by the right man in the right way... the wrong instruction will be given by the wrong man in the wrong way... there is no one simple answer unless it is what is important is the choice of the teacher, and the choice of him who chooses the teacher.'(3)

'There are teachers who represent rebellion against the social mores of our time: those who would remove all constraints in the area of sex and preach liberation and encourage young girls to have 5 condoms in their handbag when they go out at night...'(4)

Lord Clifford of Chudleigh pursued the accusation further still by revealing that moral subversion is a weapon of a broader orchestrated political attack on the foundation of British society. Moreover, this subversion takes a very special form: the 'creation' of young homosexuals:

> 'the International Socialists and their allies are responsible for many
> of the more notorious cases of sexual mal education (Little Red
> Schoolbook)... encouragement of young to rebel against their
> parents'...'Surely the most obvious of all ways in which to write off
> a country is to persuade children to become homosexual- and what
> better chance of doing this is there than to let Gay Liberation reach
> a child when he or she is going through that stage?... The National
> Council for Civil Licence - as it should be called - sponsors the
> Children's Rights Campaign with its anti-parent anti-authority
> emphasis... Have parents no rights? Are they to be ridden roughshod
> over by the trendy educational fringe?'(5)(6)

Such amateur sexology will appear again, particularly in the 1986 debate, at which time legislative steps are considered to counter this 'threat'. Baroness Gaitskell attempted to inject reason back into the debate, bringing it back to the essential issue:

> 'While parents have not had enough responsibility, teachers have
> been given a responsibility for which they are not qualified, and so
> we have a terrible mess in certain aspects of this subject.'(7)

Elles agreed that education in sexuality and relationships differs qualitatively from the other examinable subjects on the school curriculum because it carries within it a political message. It is recognised by both 'progressives' and 'traditionalists' that to restrict sex education to biological functions would be to teach no more than 'sex', which would be to violate the integrity of sexuality within human relationships. However, this raises the question of what kind of education is suited to the transmission of knowledge in this respect. The simplistic traditionalist formula is to attach to biological facts a set of conventional values to which it is morally 'correct' and desirable to conform. The alternative progressive educational formula is to subject to critical examination the historical relations between the sexes *as a means* of deciding what are correct values.

But this is a dangerous direction, involving as it does analysis of the status of women, and in turn the question of sexual 'rights' and 'responsibilities' to sexual expression, to one's own body etc. Such education must end with discussion of what is 'acceptable' sexuality, itself - something traditionalists do not believe suited to school education. In one sense, teachers who are conscientious enough to fulfil their obligations to sex education are forced into such a choice and towards the controversy which can follow exposure of such classroom discussion. Elles was aware that teachers have access to a form of political education through this subject, but like her colleagues, has no clear solution to what she regarded as the problem. This Lords debate in one sense grappled with the question of what kind of sex education is it permissible for teachers to teach, which does not open the 'Pandora's Box' of a form of political education which is anathema to conservative thinking.

On the other hand, most of those who are critical of what they regard (or fantasise) as excessively 'libertarian' sex education equally recognise that they cannot dispense with the services of teachers. What they feel is necessary is a suitable 'policing' mechanism with which to exercise control over teachers. For it is recognised that sex education in schools is required to promote the health and welfare of pupils, and that parents as a whole have not shown themselves able to fulfil totally this task. Furthermore, it is also recognised that school children need to be taught a set of standard values by which they may judge the amorality and 'packaged' sexuality to which they are increasingly exposed in the media of a free-enterprise society.

Searching for a solution to this dilemma, some of the honourable members identified a policing mechanism, Elles choosing the head teacher as the person ultimately responsible for teachers' behaviour, Lord Clifford preferring the solution of a compulsory working relationship between parents and teachers:

> 'strong parent-teacher association, careful and open staff consultation and parent consultation. This obviates untrained and unacceptable teachers taking on the job. The parents simply would not allow it. While there must be a balance in education between the wishes of parents and society, not enough attention is paid to consultation...which has produced doubt and mistrust...In independent schools the head teacher loses his job if the parents rebel, but in the state school the teacher is a secure as a bishop... sex education in state schools must be in the hands of the right teachers, and the subject matter must be agreed by the parent-teacher association... parents' rights can be best protected by a strong parent-teacher association...In this day and age, sex education is not a separate educational discipline... It seems to me that in these circumstances parents' rights can be best protected by a mandatory strong parent-teacher association. If there had been some prior consultation there would not have been the trouble which we had in Exeter when the educational authority made some ham-fisted reference to teaching homosexual relations.'(8)

The weakness in both proposals stems from the absence of any nationally-recognised procedure for the creation of a sex education curriculum over which parents, teachers and head teachers can decide on preferences. The burden is placed instead upon the head teacher and staff to draw upon some preferred but acceptable approach as a starting point. However, the independent character of the educational system will necessitate the creation of as many curricula as there are schools, drawn from a wide variety of independent commercial and local authority sources. Traditionalist-leaning head teachers will insist on the provision of a corresponding sex education curriculum; 'progressive'-leaning head teachers will act accordingly. The Lords' attempt to confront the problem of choice of content in sex education, and responsibility for it, failed to address the full complexity of the matter. While conservatives have traditionally upheld the local autonomy of schools as a bastion against left-wing mass political education, within this subject (where a standard curriculum is lacking), local school autonomy is the very means by which many examples of progressive sex education have been able to emerge, to the chagrin of the right. And this does not stop head teachers and teachers turning to organisations for curriculum assistance which the right does not approve of. In particular, the FPA manifesto gave some 'traditionalists' cause for alarm:

> '...(An objective of sex education should be the provision of)... an incentive to work towards a society in which archaic sex laws, irrational fears of sex and sexual exploitation are non-existent.'(9)

For the traditionalist this places the FPA firmly in the ranks of suspect sex reform movements, disqualifying it as a contributor to state education of the young (interpreted as the process by which an understanding and appreciation of 'ideal' moral values is acquired. The FPA was also condemned as an unsuitable organisation to be responsible for sex education training by the very nature of its endorsement of contraceptives as a means of controlling unwanted pregnancies. In this respect the fundamental divisions between the traditionalist and progressive educational perspectives are at their sharpest: the former founded on the principle that education should be about the control of hedonistic tendencies, as this classic portrayal of what is regarded as progressive sex education reveals:

> 'We tell them what a unique and wonderful thing sex is, and having instructed them as best we possibly can on how at the same time both to copulate but not to procreate, is it not surprising that the children then go and try it out ?.... Mistakes are made. More pregnancies ensue, and so the vicious circle starts again, leaving a trail of scarred emotions and bruised even ruined lives in its wake.'(10)

Earl Ferrers condemned what he believed was the 'progressive' sex education position because of its attitude to marriage and responsible contraceptive practice:

> 'Instruction is given for partners, inferring... that such unions will be outside the context of marriage....It is debasing to infer that to use contraceptives is responsible without making it plain that promiscuity which contraceptives inevitably encourage is socially irresponsible.'

> 'It is dishonest (for the FPA *et al.*) to teach or to claim that contraception is safe, either for pregnancy or health... 'Play safe, ask your chemist for contraceptives'.....(this) correlates sexual intercourse with playing or commendable relaxation....safe from what? Pregnancy? This is not so, disease, that certainly is not so, reprimand? Emotional upheaval... they do not say anything about that.'(11)

The differences in attitude to sexuality and 'right' behaviour are profound and based partly upon strongly held philosophical differences about the place of sexual pleasure in life. For the FPA, the contraceptive 'benefits' to the threat of pregnancy in adolescence and beyond outweigh the 'costs' for practical as well as philosophical reasons. Thus, it may draw upon evidence to argue that responsible sexual attitudes and behaviour cannot be created by means of fear, ignorance or repression. It has also defended the 'contraceptive option' because of its unwillingness to approach adolescent sexuality negatively because of the consequences of such a portrayal for emotional and attitudinal development in later life.

The traditionalist position reverses the cost-benefit ratio, challenging not only the evidence used by the FPA to support its position, but its right to present itself as an authority in this field, in spite of the bona fide status given to it by the government Ministry of Health. In the absence of a universally-accepted scientific orthodoxy on which the 'progressive' movements can base their approaches, organisations such as the FPA are portrayed as covert 'fifth-columnists' in schools. *This critical failure to reach a working consensus on even the most fundamental principles which should underlie a school curriculum lies at the root of the continuing crisis of sex education in Britain.* However the vacuum works to the detriment to those of 'progressive' and 'traditionalist' persuasions alike. In the absence of any established minimum principles or regulations for teaching content and practice, traditionalists have no more means to prevent teachers from turning to the FPA for guidance than progressives have to take steps to end sex education based on 'repressive' principles.

For this reason, in spite of her demands for an alternative form of teaching, Baroness Elles was forced into the position she herself accepted to be unsatisfactory: the right of parents to withdraw their children from classes they do not approve of (recognising that the child can pay dearly for missing such lessons, and the inability of many families to take advantage of moving to another district with a preferred school). Failing all else, she noted that it is well to recall that there is no statutory obligation on head teachers to provide sex education at all.

The Role of Government in 1976

By the end of the 1976 debate, the Lords had aired the major issues, and took the first steps towards identifying the course of action which would be substantially advanced in 1986. This course of action had two parts: firstly there was the identification of the basic values on which all school sex education curricula should be constructed; and secondly, identification of the source of authority which could ensure that these values are recognised and respected by all of those concerned with education.

Coming to the defence of the FPA, Baroness Gaitskell recognised the need for a mechanism by which basic working principles could be established, under government supervision:

'and the FPA believes that sex educators have a responsibility to be trained..[and]... has started a training course in this field. I think that sex education should be an important part of teacher training colleges and not dealt with just by the Health Education Council or even the Marriage Guidance Council..The Department of Education and Science should set up a committee or council of social workers who specialise in this subject for the curriculum.'(12)

The Lord Bishop of Norwich, supporting the traditionalist position, believed that schools should be guided by the attitudes in the community around them, and in particular the 'Christian insights which can lead towards a permanent marriage relationship'. However, he insisted that it is the responsibility of national government to add its authority to this foundation, something it has persistently refused to do. Lord Longford added that while:

'governments have rightly shied away from pontificating on morals...I submit that it is impossible to provide a sex education which does not impart values of some kind, positive or negative; in other words, sex education which does not place sex in a moral context teaches immorality.'(13)

Recognising that, however vital to local consensus and confidence, the efforts of parent-teacher associations cannot replace the need for *national* guidelines on which they can draw direction, Lord Lauderdale takes Longford's point to its natural conclusion. With some persistence the Lord demanded an answer to the question:

> 'Does the government provide guidelines for the sex education curriculum, and if so what advice is given to teachers on the subject of chastity and fidelity... Does the government agree that sex education must be coupled with instruction in right and wrong in the principle of chastity before marriage... [persisting]... [as the government is able to give advice on the curriculum]... Is it taught that things are right and wrong?'(14)

Crowther-Hunt finally provided a full and revealing answer:

> 'I have not so far tried to define what I mean by sex education, or to consider the questions of who should teach it, when it is best for the first teaching to be given, or where teachers stand on giving moral guidance to their pupils...I have no powers to prescribe the details of the curriculum in schools in England, and my Department's role in curriculum development is limited to giving advice and providing channels for the exchange of information... local education authorities are taking advantage of the increasing wealth of teaching material and expertise which is available... Her Majesty's Inspectors play an extensive part in exchange of information' [through] conferences with the Association of Teachers.'(15)

This questioning causes Crowther-Hunt no small problem, for two reasons: firstly, for reasons of political expediency, no government had been willing to offer prescriptions for moral education during the post-war period, when so many moral and educational assumptions were subjected to critical revision. Secondly, Crowther-Hunt's evasions suggest that the (Labour) government of the day had some sympathy with the 'progressive' spirit in education in general, and preferred to 'sub-contract' the task of developing the principles and practice of this nascent subject to the semi-autonomous government-funded organisations such as the Schools Council, along with 'bona fide' independent organisations such as the FPA. Appreciating that this approach is no longer regarded as satisfactory by his interrogators, Crowther-Hunt was compelled to adopt the following pragmatic defence of the Government position:

> '...what is taught in schools about attitudes and values will be influenced and substantially so by the attitudes and values prevalent

in society as a whole...it will always be immensely difficult to identify specific actions or methods which will influence pupils in their moral attitudes. Each generation will come to its own conclusions, drawing on its own environment including the formal consent of the school curriculum but also including at least equally potent other influences.'(16)

With this, the traditionalist Lords abandon their cross-examination and the 1976 debate comes to a close, the FPA remaining (financially) unscathed. What the Minister appears to be saying here is that teachers can only be guided by the status quo in the sex education they offer, which by implication is in constant flux, or by what they feel is likely to be *persuasive to pupils*. If this interpretation is correct, it suggests an underlying affinity of the government Ministry of Education with the 'progressive' thinking of the day which failed to establish sufficient support within British society as a whole to survive the 1980s.

Sex Education in the 1986 Education Act

It has been suggested so far that government unwillingness to concede measures to balance out the influence of the 'progressive' or liberalising tendency characterised the development of moral education for schools during the 1960s and 1970s. However this broadly-based movement, which pioneered moral learning programmes believed to be suited to the times, never explicitly established the basic principles on which its curricula were to be further developed, beyond a vague desire to dismantle the repressive educational approach to sexual morality inherited from the Victorians. More importantly, this movement failed to win over sufficient educational and health professionals, politicians and parents of conservative leaning to the idea that sex education could be taught in schools in a more positive manner, leading to more responsible sexual behaviour among the young. This stemmed in part from differences of approach to sex education within the progressive tendency itself which could not easily be reconciled, rooted in the broader political push for sexual reform and defence of the rights of sexual minorities.

The progressive movement had not succeeded in consolidating a guide to sex education curriculum planning which incorporated elements of the new sexual politics (including the needs of sexual minority groups) suitable for adolescent education, while retaining a moral framework which would accommodate or avoid alienating the 'middle-ground' of traditionalist thinking. Consequently, although rather helpless to do much about it at the national level during the 1970s, traditionalists were able to hold up literally any commercial product connected with 'sex education' as an example of the amoral libertarianism which was being imported by Left-leaning teachers into the classroom, the much villified 'Make it Happy' by Jane Cousins was to the 1980s what the 'Little Red Schoolbook' was to the 1970s. Moreover, it might fairly be said that progressives in sex education were in no position to know what was being taught in their name. Consequently, school sex education has remained the victim of a continuous stream of media scandals, both real and imaginary.

During the 1970s, the impasse over what should constitute sex education remained in the form of an enmity between progressive and traditionalist interest groups. What changed this situation dramatically by the mid-1980s was the ascendancy of Conservative Party power.

Here was established a power base for the re-assertion of traditionalist educational thinking. Conservative politics, among other things, was determined to roll back socialistic measures introduced into the educational system in a number of ways, one being paradoxically, the announcement of a move towards a national core curriculum, promising to end the autonomy of the single school on curriculum matters. The political platform of a Conservative Party elected to a third term in 1986 contained a commitment to reinforce 'traditional Victorian morality', both in public life (eg. the media) and in the classroom. An obvious focus for this promised moral 'counter-revolution' was school sex education.

Parliamentary representatives of the traditionalist tendency set out to reduce the power of bureaucracies and independent organisations which had attracted into their ranks progressive educational advisers (given the epithet 'experts' used in a derogatory way) on moral and sexual matters. Local Education Authorities, whose task, among other things, was to undertake curriculum development research on behalf of schools are seen as one locus of this tendency. Conservatives depend upon an assumption that parents and head teachers are more likely to be supportive of 'traditional values' than the teaching profession as a whole. This being so, making use of its populist appeal, the Government sought to expand parent representation on school governing bodies through the 1980 *Educational (Amendment) Act* .

In March 1986, both Houses returned to the subject of school sex education within a second reading of the Education Bill (the first time since 1976). Though with a largely different cast from 1976, the debates which ensued revealed remarkably similar prejudices and questionable assumptions on both sides, with more evident party political antagonism showing through in the Commons. Although a knee jerk party-political bullishness on both sides clouded the issues which had to be confronted rationally, the germs of solutions voiced in 1976 are also more clearly articulated, mainly by the traditionalist lobby, which alone showed a willingness to grasp the nettle of curriculum *values*.

The Bill was introduced by the Earl of Swinton:

> 'The Bill deals with school government... the aim is to re-establish
> school governing bodies... The 1944 Act established the governing
> framework (to give the school an individual life of its own). It is
> exactly those principles which this Bill pursues for the vision of the
> 1944 Act did not become a reality... domination by LEAs: appointees
> with obscure powers... failure to harness parents natural interest in
> childrens' progress... schools have become mere adjunct to the LEA.
> The 1980 Act provided a valuable step forward by ending the
> practice of grouping many schools under a single governing body
> and by introducing elected parent and teacher governors. The present
> Bill will complete the process removing power of LEAs to appoint
> most of the governors... no interest will predominate... The clauses
> require that the LEAs state their curricular policy for all the schools
> in the area... it will then be for the governing body to state its policy
> for the curriculum in the school, finally the head teacher's role is
> explicit by allocating to him the determination and organisation of
> the curriculum. Clauses 24 and 25 contain significant provisions
> which will enable all parents, not just the minority who become
> parent governors, to become more involved in the work of the
> school... need to involve pupils as well as teachers on equal
> basis.'(17)

The alarms sounded in 1976 over the political import of sex education and
the motives of those mandated to conduct this education are responded to here
in a re-balancing of power over curriculum content which in theory will permit
an alliance of head teachers and parent governors to police any excesses of
teachers and their advisers. The measure is a shrewd one on the part of the
government not least because it manages at this stage to remain at a safe
distance from the thorny problems of curriculum content, which must be
shouldered by the above alliance. Parents in particular will have to take a
greater responsibility for their childrens' sex education, and any attendant
problems which arise henceforth. One assumes either that the Government
believed that the moral predilection of the two parties is sufficient to the task
of confronting these issues; or that the background knowledge or competence
required to fulfil this task will be acquired 'on the way'. Whatever, the case,
there is a sense that the contributions of all and sundry NGOs will no longer
be so required in future, nor their idea of a morality which could be modified
according to changes in the status quo.

The government was not to get off so easily, however, as traditionalists in its
own ranks recalled that the 1976 debate had already concluded that curriculum
direction must come from the highest authority for it to be effective. An

amendment put forward by Viscount Buckmaster (representing the position of, among others, the conservative interest group 'Family and Youth Concern' (Responsible Society), aimed to pin down head teachers and parents even more firmly to a strict traditional code:

'It shall be the duty of every LEA and head teacher be responsible to ensure that any sex education materials used in schools do not advocate any illegal act or act of obscenity, and any such teaching shall comply with the religious and moral beliefs of the parents of the children at the school and shall be given in the context of enduring family life. [Secondly] It shall be the right of every parent to be informed in advance of the content of any sex education to be given at the school and notwithstanding the provisions of subsection 1 above it shall be the right of any parent to withdraw his child from any sex education to which that parent objects.'(18)

Not willing to be pushed by its own right-wing into measures which would have disruptive and unworkable consequences for the very individuals groomed for this new burden, the government ('though sympathetic') could not agree to such an amendment, holding as it does the prospect of compulsory vetting of every piece of sex education material. Whether they welcomed the prospect or not, traditionalists would have to continue to rely upon the teaching profession:

'to exercise good judgement in planning their teaching and selecting appropriate teaching materials... subject to the regulations and to the pressure parents can exert at their annual meetings.'(19)

Taking on the 1976 mantle of Baroness Elles, Baroness Cox conceded that the new proposals for parental involvement stand or fall in practice on the degree to which they respond to this new responsibility in such numbers as to be representative of the whole community. This is highly significant in its recognition that the weakness of the progressive claim to sex education stemmed from its failure to secure sufficient political, professional and public sympathy and support for the approaches it advocated:

'The increased involvement of parents as governors is to be warmly welcomed... However, these changes will be effective only if parents are willing to come forward for election and actively participate in discussions and decisions. It is profoundly to be hoped that politically motivated parents of any political allegiance will not organise 'caucuses' or 'slates' to achieve the kind of partisan or politicised ambience that this legislation is intended to remove... I should like to see provision made for the wider dissemination of information about schools, especially their budgets and curricula to any parents or members of the public who wish to receive it.'(20)

What this government was willing to consider, in contrast to that of 1976, was an amendment from its traditionalist ranks which secures government-legal endorsement of a moral orientation for all attempts to develop sex education curricula. In an alarmist style which recalls the more outrageous claims of 1976, Lord Buckmaster prefaced his proposal with information that:

'A great deal of sex education today, particularly in our maintained schools is amoral if not downright immoral, dealing as it does with no element of moral guidance... indeed the theme running through most of this literature is that sexual activity among teenagers of whatever age is quite normal and natural and also quite harmless provided one takes appropriate precautions to avoid pregnancy or a sexually transmitted disease...'(21)

Referring to what is probably the most widely used sex education resource manual in British schools: *Taught Not Caught* (22), Buckmaster claimed:

'there is a series of projects for children of nine upwards in which various methods are used to persuade children that there are no rights and wrongs, that they must make their own minds up who they have sex with and when, and that parents are oppressors to be circumvented... there is an obsession to persuade young people to regard homosexual relationships as being in everyway as acceptable as others...'(23)

Baroness Cox added her own example:

'On moral education, there is widespread concern about the recent developments in the teaching of sex education particularly under the rubric of so called anti-sexism. Too often this is used to attack the concepts of traditional family life and of heterosexuality. The recent edition of 'Teaching London Kids' which is written by teachers in London schools specifically advocates the promotion of gay issues in the school curriculum... One teacher claims she tries to use her opportunities as a teacher to undo the damage caused by the conditioning process which makes children regard heterosexuality as the real world... deeply offensive to many parents... I cannot imagine how on earth in this age of AIDS we can be contemplating gay issues in the curriculum.'(24)

Having the government counter themes which he believed to be running through contemporary education ('that homosexual relations are just as acceptable as heterosexual relations; that there is nothing basically wrong with under-age sex provided one takes the appropriate precaution; and that incest can on occasions be regarded as a loving relationship') (25), Lord Buckmaster moved Amendment 53:

> 'Such sex education as is given in schools shall have due regard to moral considerations and the promotion of stable family life.'(26)

Airing doubts about the value of legislating on morality, Lord Denning believed, nevertheless, that legal status is required to give weight to a principle which is believed must stand above the curriculum decision-making process at the local level. The Lord Bishop of London was clear about the import of this amendment if accepted:

> 'it is not simply a general statement of principle or a moral exhortation; it is actually a requirement that sex education should be given in a particular context.'(27)

The amendment was accepted, albeit with removal of the word 'stable' from 'family life' - a problem which will be raised when the Commons have the opportunity to discuss the matter. Baroness Hooper, for the Government, summed up:

> '...Teaching about the physical aspects of sexuality cannot however in the government's view, be seen in isolation and must be set within a wider moral context of an education system which encourages young people to understand the importance of self-restraint, self-respect and respect for others; and also lays the foundations for loving and caring relationships and a stable family life... When so much which children see around them in their everyday lives- in the media, in advertising and regrettably sometimes in the behaviour of their elders- appears to cheapen and devalue the concept of lasting and meaningful relationships and to disregard questions of moral values it is difficult but schools can play an important role. Pupils should acquire the necessary knowledge, skills and qualities of character needed to make responsible choices about their own lifestyles both now and as adults.'(28)

The Reaction of the House of Commons(29)

In the ensuing debate on the Bill in the House of Commons, both Labour and Liberal Members of Parliament rushed to the defence of the educational status quo; that is, what they believed to be 'progressive' sex education, and to the right of teachers to pursue their own interpretation of this. As in 1976, the debate addressed simultaneously two distinct issues: the desired content of sex education; and the mechanism through which this content should be decided and monitored in implementation in the classroom. It is remarkable (though predictable, historically speaking)(30) that, in the final analysis, a large part of the debate on the theory and practice of school sex education in Britain continues to hinge upon attitudes to *homosexuality*.

Concerning the first issue, shadow education minister, Giles Radice dismissed the principle and practice of government involvement out of hand, with an unconvincing claim that to his knowledge the subject is always taught in a sensible manner.(31)

Joining this counter-attack, Liberal, Clement Freud objected to 'family life' being placed on a moral pedestal for the strange reason that not all children have access to such an existence, and may thereby be disadvantaged. He is perhaps on firmer ground when voicing the suspicion that:

> 'As for 'the value of family life', I think we all know the sorts of families that those who inserted the clause had in mind. They constitute a decreasing proportion of contemporary families and should not be given a sort of class one treatment in respect of children, because that effectively relegates all other types of families to class three or four or worse... It is an undisputed fact that British children are more naive about sex education than children in Scandinavia. But putting this right can only be achieved by good practice not by defective legislation.'(32)

Mr D E Thomas attempted to expose the intolerance of the amendment, arguing that it is no less than:

> 'a form of propaganda for heterosexuality... However we must accept and understand the issues of homosexuality, lesbianism and other varied sexual preferences in a tolerant society.'(33)

Comparing the reactions of critics of the government amendment, it is difficult to avoid comparing their uncompromising tone with the melodramatic revelations of subversive sex education by traditionalists; such are the emotions generated by this subject within Parliament. This is all the less excusable considering the fact that those seeking to defend the cause of progressive sex education in this arena succeed merely to expose its weaknesses.

In seeking to respond to the demands of its traditionalist supporters, the government has sought to elevate to a prime position, within school education, the uncontestable principle of the value of lasting relationships - particularly where dependents are involved ('the family'). Whether by accident or design, this principle can be interpreted to accommodate homosexual as well as heterosexual relations; though to his credit only (Conservative) Steve Norris is willing to enter the middle ground between the party positions to raise this fact.(34) This, however, is not what the majority of its supporters intended. For example Conservative, Rumbold believed that:

> 'it will go much of the way to ensuring that irresponsible and unrepresentative teaching does not find its way into the classroom... blocking... educationally unsound teaching materials and methods, and the propagation of extreme and unrepresentative views of sexual ethics... [it constitutes] a clear statement of broad principles.'(35)

By contrast, opposition critic Mr Thomas was unwilling to concede any meaning to this amendment other than outright discrimination against homosexuals. In light of the above, it may be argued that such argumentation was unlikely to serve the cause of homosexuality, merely confirming the traditionalist's worst fears: that the 'Left' wishes to promote in the classroom *short-term* sexual liaisons of either a homosexual or heterosexual kind, depending on one's preference. This kind of response also encourages traditionalistic expressions of angst over sexual orientation which has the effect merely of distorting course of the debate. Thus, the subject of homosexuality recurred repeatedly with increasingly exotic examples; Conservatives, Batiste and Bruinvels, respectively:

> 'I have another document that has been produced by the Bradford and Leeds lesbian teachers group. Mention has been made of the need to be sensitive towards the problems of homosexual teachers. I accept that but I do not think that I am alone in finding blatant proselytising by homosexual groups in schools unacceptable and offensive. This document states: "At every level of the educational system students are misinformed about lesbians and denied the opportunity to explore anything other than a very conventional heterosexual relationship. Young women are forcibly directed and channelled into heterosexuality"... It is indeed a very sad day if heterosexuality has become a crime.'(36)

> 'I fear that mentioning these subjects at such an early age will tempt a child to find out more and put into practice at an early age what is best left to a much later age if one has to go down that dubious path.'(37)

In similar fashion, the focus upon the family may be interpreted as a disguised attempt to give national-legal approval to the traditional paternalistic version against other arrangements, as Freud insisted. *However, it need not have been interpreted in this way*, but regarded as a landmark step from which progressives as well as traditionalists may work toward broadly agreed principles for practice. To ignore this implication, as Clement Freud did in declaring the amendment to be the work of the 'moral or loony right'(38) was to do the cause of sex education a great disservice. For doubts about what does or should constitute school sex education are sincerely held, and eloquently expressed by Conservative, Bruinvels:

> 'To me sex education is fast becoming a mass of conflicting ideas and ideologies. If we knew what sex education was about, we could understand its meanings and perhaps matters would not be as worrying as they are... Gone are the days of plain biology... some teachers [now] promote their own sexual preferences, prejudices and proclivities... in such a way as to encourage very young children to accept as abnormal what we think is normal and vice versa... We must ask ourselves what is the purpose of sex education in schools. I do not totally oppose it, but who should give that form of education? Are the teachers qualified? Are they specialists? Does sex education come within the overall syllabus of any particular department? Should it not be included purely and exclusively in biology? What is the content of sex education? Should it be all-inclusive with moral teaching, a social setting, biological facts and medical information? At what age should pupils come forward to be taught?... I should like teachers to be totally qualified in the sex education that they are giving, but many have no experience.'(39)

Cormack returned to national standardisation as the only formula to resolve the impasse:

> 'The only way to deal with this matter properly and sensibly is for the Government not to abdicate their responsibilities, but to grasp the opportunities and realise that, in effect, there must be an agreed syllabus... It is the facts that must be taught... against an accepted background. [However]... in this country the overwhelming majority of people believe that normal family life consists of two parents, who are married with children. This is the background against which the facts must be taught... If the parents believe otherwise it is for them to teach what some of us might regard as dangerous deviations... We need an agreed syllabus; we need parents throughout the land to feel that their children can go to school and be taught the facts - many of them dangerous facts - without overtones, without insinuations, without moral or immoral indoctrination'(40)

The question of agreement over the *content* of school sex education being only part of the problem, Members turned their attention to the appropriate *mechanism* through which this content should be decided and monitored in theory and practice. Here there was agreement in principle but disagreement in detail. The shadow education spokesman, Radice, was in no doubt that:

> 'There is nothing in the Bill that will help to ensure that all local authorities provide adequate minimum standards of provision... I do not believe that a general clause of this kind helps to ensure that sex education is properly taught in schools. Is this not a matter that could be better dealt with by the Secretary of State's inspectors, who could issue proper advice and ensure that it was carried out?'(41)

Elsewhere he proposed a structure for curriculum planning in the form of 'a partnership involving teachers, parents, governing bodies and local education authorities', therefore avoiding the need for legislation.(42) Baroness Hooper agreed that legislation is inappropriate:

> 'Her Majesty's Inspectorate of schools will also be offering substantive professional guidance on the teaching of sex education... "Health Education from 5 to 16 Years". These are the appropriate vehicles for the detailed content of sex education provision... not primary legislation.'(43)

However, Minister of Education, Christopher Patten insisted that it is right and proper for central government to 'give a lead to LEAs and schools' in the form of this amendment. By implication, this is a recognition by Parliament that the advisory deliberations of HMIs carry insufficient authority to influence practice nationally. Nor, in spite of the confidence expressed by Hooper or Radice, do existing HMI documents actually offer the kind of detailed guidelines they are supposed to be 'appropriate vehicles' for (see chapter 4).

The principal recipient of the legislative directive is to be neither the LEA nor school but the *school governing body* (in particular, head teachers working with parent 'representatives'). In the Lords debate of the 30th October 1986, Baroness Hooper had made clear that school governors would henceforth be responsible for deciding whether sex education should be given in the school and, if so, what should be its content and organisation. This would include decisions upon the kinds of textbooks and teaching, and how controversial issues should be tackled. In the Lords, Baroness Cox had been concerned that parental involvement would be corrupted through the cooption of partisan opinion of the Gillick variety. In the Commons debate, McKay even doubted the capacity of school governors as a whole to undertake the tasks set for them by the government:

'I am sure that the Secretary of State is aware that the governors of schools do not work with regard to such practicalities. In practice, governors only meet four times per year - that is, if they are lucky. They do not always turn up to all four meetings so why put the responsibility on governors when we have an honourable teaching profession?' (44)

However, the final word must go to Norris for perceiving that the task of standardising detailed curriculum guidelines for such a controversial subject must be taken on by a *national* authority, working in consultation with, and with the confidence of local structures such as governors:

'The only practical solution to the degree of parental and Parliamentary concern which has been expressed tonight and on other occasions is to consider that circular (DES) as the *basis for a comprehensive code of practice*. It should be the duty and obligation of local authorities to have regard to it. It specifies the variety of subjects to be involved and what responsible teachers should be teaching and the kind of material to be used... members should have grave reservations about the idea that the problem will be solved by giving the responsibility to the governors.' (45)

Conclusion

In 1976, the House of Lords expressed a variety of anxieties about the contemporary state of British school sex education. These anxieties stemmed in part from an admitted ignorance over the content and style of teaching which was taking place in schools. This feeling of ignorance re-surfaced again in the 1986 Education Bill debates in both Houses.

Both debates revealed that lack of knowledge of the details of school practice creates a situation in which senior decision-makers can be influenced by rumour, distortions of facts and allegations of bad practice, and that this has been a direct consequence of the ad hoc manner in which schools have been encouraged to introduce sex education in to the curriculum. What is significant is that the legislative events of 1986 generated debates which forced the honourable Members of both Houses to gain a far sharper perception of the problems which must be resolved for a constructive political management of state sex education to be feasible, even if the ideological dimension remains tainted by an homophobia and expressed distrust of sections of the teaching profession. Nevertheless, it is recognised that this issue can only be resolved with *acceptable* national mechanisms of control which the majority of teachers would support.

As in other European countries which have confronted this subject seriously, Parliament has begun to recognise the necessity of dealing with the ideological content and political management of state school sex education in a single approach, as the two are inextricably connected. This appeared in the debates above in the form of a series of what might be called 'anxiety areas', each of which requires a structural as well as ideological recipe for their resolution. These areas are addressed systematically against the background of European strategies in the concluding chapter.

Notes

1. Davies, C 'Moralists, Causalists, Sex, Law and Morality' in Armytage, W, Chester, R and Peel, J eds *Changing Patterns of Sexual Behaviour* Academic Press 1980, p 41.)

2. *Parliamentary Debates:* House of Lords Official Report (Hansard) Vol 367 No18 14th January 1976, HMSO cols 136-7

3. ibid. col 178

4. ibid. col 204

5. ibid. col 237

6. ibid. col 238

7. ibid. col 180

8. ibid. cols 238/240

9. Baroness Elles quoting Freda Parker, founder of the FPA Education Unit. ibid. col 139

10. ibid. col 171

11. ibid. cols 173ff

12. ibid. col 180

13. ibid. col 193

14. ibid. cols 254ff

15. ibid. col 253.

16. ibid. col 260

17. *Education Bill*; Second Reading. House of Lords (Hansard) Official Report Vol 472 No 57 March 1986 col 442

18. *Education Bill* Vol 473 No74. April 15th 1986 col 646 49B

19. ibid. col 650

20. ibid. col 448

21. *Education Bill* House of Lords Official report Vol 475 No 97. 21 May 1986 col 225

22. The Clarity Collective *Taught Not Caught: Strategies for Sex Education* LDA Cambridge 1983

23. *Education Bill* House of Lords Vol 473 No 74 16th April 1986 col 647

24. *Education Bill* House of Lords Official Report Vol 475 No 97 21 May 1986 col 229-30

25. ibid. col 225

26. ibid.

27. ibid. col 228

28. *Education Bill* House of Lords Official Report Vol 475 No99 2 June 1986 col 569.

29. *Education Bill* House of Commons Official Report Vol 99 No 125 10 June 1986.

30. see Weeks, Jeffrey *Sex, Politics and Society* Longman Harlow 1981 chapter 6

31. *Education Bill* House of Commons *Parliamentary Debates* Tuesday 10 June 1986 Vol 99 No 125 col 198

32. *Parliamentary Debates* House of Commons Official Report of Standing Committee B *Education Bill (Lords)* 1st -10th July 1986 Part II col 442

33. *Education Bill* House of Commons *Parliamentary Debates* Tuesday 10 June 1986 Vol 99 No 125 col 230

34. *Parliamentary Debates* House of Commons Official Report of Standing Committee B *Education Bill (Lords)* 1st -10th July 1986 Part II col 445

35. House of Commons Official Debate *Parliamentary Debates* Wed 22 October 1986 Vol 102 No 160 col 1056

36. *Parliamentary Debates* House of Commons Official Reports vol 99 No 125 Tuesday 10th June 1986 col 238

37. *Parliamentary Debates* House of Commons Official Report Vol 102 No 160 22nd October 1986 col 1065

38. *Parliamentary Debates* House of Commons Official Report of Standing Committee B *Education Bill (Lords)* 1st -10th July 1986 Part II col 442

39. House of Commons Official Debate *Parliamentary Debates* Wed 22 October 1986 Vol 102 No 160 col 1064

40. ibid. col 1086

41. *Parliamentary Debates* House of Commons Official Reports Vol 99 No 125 10th June 1986 col 197

42. House of Commons Official Debate *Parliamentary Debates* Wed 22 October 1986 Vol 102 No 160 col 1062.

43. ibid. col 1060

44. ibid. col 1082

45. ibid. col 1081

Chapter 3

Fact and Value in the Knowledge Base of Sex Education

In the 1976 House of Lords debate on school sex education, Baroness Elles made a distinction between the teaching of history and geography 'which are concerned with the imparting of information and the extension of knowledge', and what she saw as the more serious business of teaching sex education, 'which influences not only mental understanding but also has an effect on patterns of behaviour, social attitudes, emotional experience... [that is]... moral education'.(1)

The statement is a useful starting point to examine the problematical relationship between facts and values in British sex education, which has yet to be resolved. Controversies reported in the media largely focus upon the moral import of presentation of 'facts' about sexuality. This has reached the point where it has been felt necessary to resort to legislation to enforce the 'correct' way of presenting 'facts' about homosexuality.(2) In matters of sex education, some feel that 'knowledge' alone has the power to corrupt. As a result, parental and other forms of consultation are used to ensure that factual information is handled by teachers in acceptable ways.(3) While parents have a right to know how and with what effect factual information about sexuality is conveyed to their children, what prospect is there of teachers relying upon a scientifically- established knowledge base for this subject without simultaneously becoming engaged in a debate over its moral import?

Elles' statement introduced a Parliamentary debate in which the competence of (certain) school teachers to undertake sex education in schools began to be seriously challenged. This challenge has created a crisis of confidence in the way schools choose to manage this subject, among those defending traditional principles of education, which shows no sign of being resolved. It is also unfortunate that the special significance attributed to this subject over others belies the fact that, according to what research exists, its quality and quantity continues to vary widely, and has an (increasingly) uncertain place in the school curriculum, in contrast to the range of examined subjects.(4) Sex education is occasionally given prominence by the media. However, this more often takes the form of 'exposés' of 'unacceptable' teaching than constructive discussion about ways and means of improving provision, integration and effectiveness. A central purpose of the introduction, by the Conservative Party, of a national curriculum is to re-focus school education towards those

40

'core' subjects which are believed to create 'marketable skills', in contrast to the broader development of the personality which has been regarded as the objective of an expanded curriculum including health and sex education.

The purpose of this chapter is to investigate the reasons for this crisis of confidence. Certain teaching aids created for schools have been judged by some conservative critics as sexological forms of 'political indoctrination'.(5) It is argued here that this constitutes a misrepresentation of *attempts* by those individuals and organisations concerned to develop this subject to come to terms with fundamental changes in the scientific interpretation ('the facts') of sexuality itself. It is proposed that a resolution to this crisis will depend partly upon a broader understanding of the social implications of contemporary sexological knowledge, and the pursuit of a national consensus on how this scientific tradition can be best used to serve the purposes of school sex education.

Facts and Values in Sex Education

The 'traditionalistic' versus 'progressive' interpretations of sex education, introduced in the last chapter, are built upon opposing preferred philosophies of sexuality. Both recognise the retreat of scientific sexology from the notion of an 'instinctual' basis of sexual identity and behaviour; ascribing to some variant of socialisation or 'learning' process of socio-sexual development. However, there are fundamental differences over the significance attached to 'learned' sexual expression. Traditionalists are more concerned with the importance of 'control' over the sex drive, and its sublimation, particularly during adolescence, into other creative activities. The progressive sentiment, by contrast,tends more toward providing a positive basis for the sexual drive to emerge in humanising, socialising ways. The 'spiritual' value attached to sexuality per se will also determine opinions about the costs and benefits of contraceptives in the adolescent years.

The two tendencies do not differ in respect of their understanding of school sex education as a formal process in which moral values are addressed by means of factual instruction about reproduction and sexual behaviour. However, a profound difference has emerged concerning how this process should occur.

One, in retrospect naïve, conception of 'traditional' sex education has the teacher providing 'objective', scientific information about sexuality and reproduction to which desired values and moral code are attached in the home by parents. The conviction that adolescents would benefit by being permitted access to hitherto taboo and restricted details about sexuality and reproduction underlies early professional and governmental statements on the subject. This is still perceived by many parents, as well as politicians, as the most desirable model. (6)

A less naïve version of 'traditionalist' sex education perceives this process as the communication of a set of pre-established moral values (eg. about the proper time and place for sexual initiation; the form sexual activity should take, and the social systems within which it should take place etc.), supported where necessary by appropriate 'objective' information. It is not the business of the teacher to pursue his/her own preferred persuasions on these matters, but to conform with the curriculum established by those to whom the school is answerable: the parent, school board, Church etc. A more sophisticated version of the above might introduce scientific sexological theorising or data which appears to support the values the education is expected to convey (eg. the essential sociological benefits of the nuclear family structure to society, or the psychological benefits of monogamous relations etc.).

By contrast, 'progressive' sex education has appeared in the form of a teacher using biological and sexological knowledge to encourage 'objective' discussion of the range of moral values pertaining in a society, with a view to pupils arriving at their own opinion. A more radical version of such education may take the form of selective communication of existing biological-sexological knowledge to permit young people to acquire a deeper understanding of their own and others sexuality, and to be able to evaluate for themselves the moral status quo.

It can be argued that Baroness Elles is making a false distinction between the teaching of history and geography, defined (merely) as 'the imparting of information and the extension of knowledge', and sex education's deeper influence on moral behaviour. For, few subjects do not raise moral and political issues from which values are created. Concepts such as love and compassion, race and racism, nationalism, freedom, human rights, democracy and so on, all convey principles of 'right' and 'wrong' behaviour, which are conveyed by subjects throughout the school curriculum. It is rather a matter of *degree* whether the educational value of, for example, history versus sex education lies in the acquisition of 'knowledge' rather than 'personal development'.

Recoiling from what she regarded as the anti-social biases of those undertaking sex education, Elles called, among other things, for a more accurate representation of the *facts* pertaining to sexual well being, reproduction and contraception than that provided by certain sex educators.(7)

As a representative of traditionalist thinking on sex education, it is apparent that Elles was more concerned that, for her, the 'wrong' values were increasingly being derived from information being passed as 'fact'. In order to avoid the charge of moral indoctrination in future, how are teachers to acquaint themselves with an accurate representation of these essential facts? No subject in the school curriculum has a universally-agreed knowledge-base, though appeal to scientific criteria assists in the establishment of a working consensus on the teaching of many.

As far as sex education is concerned, there is as yet no agreed knowledge-base. This is to say that there are as many disagreements over the 'facts' of sexuality as the values which should be so derived. In spite of this state of affairs, in practice, the teacher is expected to rely upon his/her *incidental* knowledge of sexuality when the subject appears in the classroom. Parliamentarians who are critical of much sex education provision have bemoaned the absence of criteria by which teachers might be judged to be 'specialists' (as opposed to 'amateurs'?) in this field. Yet, failing to perceive anything between 'biology' and 'indoctrination', as some have claimed, they are ignoring the existence of extensive historical, biological, medical and social scientific analyses of sexuality, which are employed in as yet undefined ways.

This chapter briefly reviews the knowledge - the sum of scientific sexologies beyond reproductive biology - on which our contemporary understanding of sexuality is based. How coherent and useful is this knowledge base for the purposes of a school-based sex education, in order to fulfil the obligations schools have to offer moral guidance? To what extent can scientific knowledge about sexual behaviour, itself offer the means for a more standardised moral component of the education, which is acceptable to the majority of teachers, parents, politicians and pupils?

If sexuality is to be regarded as a phenomenon capable of some form of scientific analysis and explanation, then there exists the *possibility* of certain values being established on the basis of what is regarded as 'objective' knowledge rather than merely sectional interests or personal persuasions. If human sexuality is amenable to biological, psychological, anthropological and sociological explanation, then the means by which values are established should depend, at least in part, on a rational examination of these scientific contributions. This is not to propose that values can in some absolute way be derived from or 'created' out of scientific 'fact'; rather that the legitimacy of certain values over others should be increased by reference to scientific evidence.

The following review of the use made of sexology in sex education draws upon the historical resumes of the development of the science and perception of sexuality in the West by Jeffrey Weeks (8), and the historical literature survey of 111 British sex education texts, published between 1938 and 1983, undertaken by Geoffrey Wallis under the supervision of Alan Beattie (9) (47% written by medical professionals; 16% by psychologists, 14% by teachers, 7% by clergy, remainder by journalists, political groups etc).

Sexology and Sex Education

Following the period in which scientific inquiry replaced Christian-theological interpretation, it is possible to identify a crude 3-stage historical chronology governing our understanding of human sexuality. Following its codification as an element of individual identity, and in accord with the principles governing science from the 19th century, the first concern was with explanations of the essence of sexuality as a fixed socio-biological human entity:

'The term (sex) refers both to an act and a category of person, to a practice and a gender...The earliest usage of the term "sex" , in the sixteenth century, referred precisely to the division of humanity into the male section and the female section (that is, differences of gender). The dominant meaning today, however, and one current since the early nineteenth century, refers to physical relations between the sexes, "to have sex". The extension of the meanings of these words indicates a shift in the way that "sexuality" (the abstract noun referring to the quality of being "sexual") is understood in our culture.'(10)

The contribution of Freudian psychology in the late 19th and 20th centuries paved the way for a shift in the previously unidimensional scientific understanding of the phenomenon by providing for the possibility that at least part of one's sexuality is indeterminate or unprogrammed by biological or other natural forces. The third stage has been in this part of the 20th century by the critical social sciences, which have provided the means for dialectical analyses of sexuality as (among other things) a necessarily *social* construction.

Analyses of the most important scientific trends which have filtered into sex education, following the dominating influence of Christianity, reveal that this filtration has been selective enough to permit much British sex education to discover 'scientific' legitimation for the dominant values (relating to the status of women, the family, chastity, normality, etc) which had already been legitimised through Christian revelation. Nevertheless, the social sciences, and most recently a sophisticated interpretation of Freudian psychoanalysis by feminist thinkers, has created a scientific basis for an anti-traditionalistic sex education.

While the ancients were concerned with the question of over-indulgence, activity and passivity in sexual behaviour, we learn that *Christianity* interpreted sexuality as first and foremost a means of reproduction, to the point of disapproving of such relations purely for pleasure. This religion's regulation of the social dimension was accomplished by the 12th century with its elevation of marriage (and sexuality within it) to the status of a sacrament. Extra-marital and non-reproductive sexual behaviour (eg. homosexuality, masturbation) was therefore sinful.

In its most conservative expression, Christianity has provided a knowledge-base for 'anti-sex education': the disavowal of secular knowledge about sexuality as corrupting, in itself, to be replaced by indirect references to love and reproduction through religious allusions. In less conservative forms, Christian values provide a continuing source of legitimacy for non-denominational as well as explicitly denominational sex education comprising moral codes to guide one's entry into the sexual life. Founded on the premise of a supernaturally-ordained unchanging 'natural' order of things, Christianity perceives sexuality as potentially dangerous not only for the soul but society. The central function of sex education is to recommend self-control over the force within in order to ensure the survival of the marriage bond, the family, and by extension society itself, from collapse. The transmission of any 'factual' or secular information about reproductive biology or the social reality of sexuality is subordinated to this end.

In 'post Christian' British society, Christian values have been proposed, for historical reasons, as a basis on which sex education should be given not in spite of but because of the moral relativism which has replaced them. In the 1976 House of Lords debate, both Lord Longford and the Lord Bishop of Norwich proposed that Christian standards could be used as an 'ideal' to provide order from the confusion of competing approaches.(11) Others reject such a mediation in a secular society because of the double standard Christianity historically imposed on women (through its attitude to extra-marital pregnancy), its heterosexual absolutism, and its generally negative perception of sexual desire.

By the 19th century, *scientific sexology*, associated with the names of Krafft-Ebing, Havelock Ellis, Hirschfeld etc., had become established, mainly through the scientific method of descriptive classification of 'behaviours'. Physicians began to take the place of the clergy as authorities on sexual behaviour. The scientific method generated its own added form of sexual morality in the form of the stratification of sexuality into the 'normal' and the 'deviant', the latter interpreted as degeneracy or perversion. Weeks applauds the positive effects this formative discipline had in extending our knowledge of sexual behaviours. However, as a knowledge base for a code of sexual morality, the science had a naive and inadequate theoretical foundation:

> 'On the other hand, in its search for the 'true' meaning of sex, in its intense interrogation of sexual difference... it has contributed to the codification of a 'sexual tradition', a more or less coherent body of assumptions, beliefs, prejudices, rules, methods of investigation and forms of moral regulation which still shape the way we live our sexualities. Is sex threatening and dangerous? If we want to believe that then we can find justification not only in a particular Christian tradition but in the writings of the founding father of sexology, Krafft-Ebing. Is sex, on the other hand, a source of potential freedom, whose liberatory power is only blocked by the regressive force of a corrupt civilisation?... If so, then justification can be found in works of polemicists and 'scientists' from the 19th century to the present.'(12)

Making a claim to legitimacy in its affiliation with medicine (pathology and its treatment), scientific sexology reinforced the biological distinction between the sexes and the instinctual nature of sexual desire. Homosexuality could be re-defined in rational-liberal fashion from being a sin to being a biosocial disposition.

It is acknowledged that *Freud's* theory of the dynamic unconscious made a vital contribution to the emerging science of sexuality, though aspects of psychoanalysis as therapy retain a connection with the assumptions underlying the formal 19th century sexology. Thus the principal (though not only) Freudian interpretation sees sexuality as a 'mechanical' force within the personality which needs to be controlled by cultural rules and taboos; a 'drive' which must force its way out either in direct sexual expression, or, if blocked, in the form of perversions or neuroses. Moreover, Freud extended the concept of sexuality to children (the psychological formation of the 'normal' adult through the 3 phases of childhood sexuality), providing the ground for most subsequent child psychology. Sex educators influenced by psychology would henceforth have to consider the control and appropriate channelling of the 'sex drive', which appears earlier in life than had previously been believed, in such a way that it is not simply repressed at the expense of the psychological health of the adolescent. In addition, explanations and the social control of homosexuality could no longer be so straightforward.

In identifying the process of sexual development through childhood by stages, Freud provided a framework by which psychosexual maladjustment could be explained in terms of arrested development. Wallis has noted that in the main, sex educators' use of Freud's ideas of the family's influence on sexual development is towards as reinforcement of the status of the family, implying that normal development can only occur within its confines. (13) Child psychologist, John Bowlby's elevation of the mother-child relationship as the determining force on the child's healthy development has been used to uphold the virtues of family life and the mother role, as well as providing explanations of the causes of problem families and child psychopathology in the breakdown of the mother-child bond.

This field of applied psychology with its focus upon the significance of the mother role appears in the field of sex education in the work of the educationalist, Newsom. His assumptions were those of the sex education thinkers of the time: that women and men have marked psychological and physical differences, which should be reflected in complementary (sexual) roles:

'The future of women's education lies not in attempting to iron out their differences from men, to reduce them to neuters, but to teach girls how to grow into women.'(14)

Education should take account of the individual differences between the sexes and their social function.(15) Moreover the Newsom Report on school education is unequivocal on the moral code which should guide sex education:

'For our part we are agreed that boys and girls should be offered firm guidance on sexual morality based on chastity before marriage and fidelity within it.'(16)

The enthusiasm with which the American 'helping' professions took to post-Freudian psychological theory, in the 1950s, gave rise to a hugely influential trend in psycho- and other forms of 'therapy'. This affected the direction of the psychiatric, educational, and social work professions, and even of religious pastoral care.(17) Ever preoccupied with personal adjustment to achieve the (functionalist) happiness which benefits both the individual and society, the applied sciences of human, and in particular women's, sexuality became preoccupied with (optimal) human sexual response (eg. in the work of Masters and Johnson) and the elimination of impediments to it. Wallis locates this new concern with sexual well-being in sex education materials produced by respectable organisations, albeit aimed at older girls:

'the aim of (the National Marriage Guidance Council's) "How to Treat a Young Wife" and its successors was for women to complement their husband's physical satisfaction and so cement the marriage bond...With the publication of Chesser's "Love and Marriage" (1957), "the whole thrust of marriage guidance moved towards an appreciation of sex as a mode of sustaining and stabilising the family" (Smart 1981, pg 48). Dais' "The Sexual Responsibility of Women" described how women's sexuality had to function on these terms, for at no time during her formal or informal upbringing has she been impressed with the fact that marriage is a realm in which she has profound personal sexual responsibility (1957 pg 2). For Davis, women must learn to both satisfy and be satisfied sexually (1957 pg 88)...'(18)

From a quite different scientific realm, *zoology* and *animal biology* have also provided a wealth of material for educators concerned with what is both proper and natural human sexual behaviour. From this discipline, descriptions of animal behaviour are employed to show that apparent biological differences between male and female are universal, leading to sexual behaviour which displays the same law-like (instinctual) forms. In this way, heterosexuality alone has been awarded the status of universal biological normality; and, by extension, sexual intercourse is understood primarily as having a reproductive purpose, in which the female role is to be understood by her biological design as a repository for the male sperm:

'Using animals as a reference point for sex education has involved two approaches, of which one has been the recommended observation of mammalian mating habits, a method repeatedly extolled in state guidelines. The second has been extensively employed and is traceable through almost 40 years of sex education material. Back in 1938, a Professor of Anatomy, G W Corner began the standard descriptive journey through the sexual habits of fish, amphibia, birds and lower mammals to stress that sexuality is inherently concerned with reproduction: "In the higher class of animals, the mammals, to which the human race belongs, male animals possess a special organ (the penis) for getting sperm cells directly into the female reproductive system"... Other zoological connections appear more recently through the use of words such as "fertilization" (Richards 1963); "mating" (Picton 1980) to describe sexual activity'.(19)

More recently, an addition to the scientific contributions to sexology, with similar ideological import for any sex education so derived, has appeared in the form of sociobiology. Sociobiologists see all social phenomena as emanations of basic genetic material, from which scientific explanation of such phenomena must ultimately be drawn. Forms of sexual life have emerged to ensure the survival of the gene. Sociobiology seeks to explain the necessary and positive functions of not merely sexual division but conflicting interests. Males and females instinctively seek reproductive advantages, males seeking out as many sexual partners in order to maximise the passing on of genes to the next generation. Females, by contrast, operate in reverse in their drive to ensure the best possible genetic inheritance for future generations. The following quotation reveals the ideological thrust of any educational or social policy which sociobiology might inform:

> 'The most socially useful thing to do is not to eliminate differences any more than one should exaggerate them, but provide equal opportunity for each sex in his or her sphere..this is the least costly of choices and helps preserve the nuclear family..'the building block of nearly all human societies.'(20)

Medical biology offers further scientific material with which to legitimate educational goals aimed to affirm the rectitude of traditional sex roles. Here the consequences of the human biochemical makeup provide an alternative or underpin instinctually-grounded sexual orientation. Wallis again reveals examples of sex education which have drawn upon such material to justify a conformist view of gender roles where the male is dominant and the female passive, explaining even the 'maternal instinct' in chemical terms:

> 'Testosterone also increases masculine aggressiveness and libido (Bundesen 1952:16) and Chartham argued that the presence of oestrogen in women meant that the mother-instinct must remain a powerful motivation for a woman taking part in love-making.'(21)

Alternative evidence from the same scientific discipline has been used to contest the notion that the chemicals which operate in the physiological development of the sexes have a corresponding effect on gender roles also, thereby subordinating cultural socialisation to biology:

> 'The evidence on human females indicates no clear increase in sexual interest during ovulation. Thus one cannot logically deduce from how primate females act during ovulation how human females will act during ovulation....We also know from endocrinologists' research on levels of androgen in human males that it is difficult to predict male sexual activity levels from knowledge of hormone levels except in quite extreme cases.'(22)

The Relevance of Medical Science in Sexology and Sex Education

The interpretations placed on medical data remain at the centre of the debate over the importance of sexual relations for human well-being. The separation of sexual intercourse from reproduction, created by the development of artificial contraceptives, has had a profound effect on the value and significance attached to sexual relations, and by extension on the social structures (such as marriage) created to manage them. A by-product of contemporary contracepting societies is the phenomenon of 'recreational' sex - a subject powerfully exploited by the mass media. Consequently, much agonising about 'correct' sex education has been devoted to devising ways of salvaging a sense of sanctity for sexual relations.

One way has been to insist that teachers highlight the psychological-emotional costs of engaging lightly in sexual activity: the squandering of a whole dimension of the love relationship for the sake of short-term returns. Alternatively, 'traditionalist' exponents of sex education call for a strategy of highlighting the greater value of long-term health over sexual enjoyment; proposing that young people be acquainted in school with medical evidence of the (potential) side-effects of contraceptives, the (potential) consequences of early intercourse on later general and reproductive health, the costs in risks of disease of sexual partner change. Controversies over sex education have to a large extent revolved around competing evaluations of the medical evidence relating to sexual relations in adolescence (eg. the threat of cervical cancer). This may change according to new scientific findings or medical events (eg. the arrival of AIDS). Nevertheless, at any one time the 'evaluation' of such relations (in the moral as well as physical 'cost-benefit' sense) can and should make reference to the broader 'objective' processes of statistical and other scientific analysis.

The Impact of Sociology

Sociological research since the 1950s has been used to challenge the validity of scientific explanations of the fixed character of the sex roles and the status these explanations attached to a single type of sexual behaviour. Moreover, *critical social theory* has provided the means to charge that much conventional scientific evidence is thinly disguised ideology used to legitimise one pattern of sexuality against possible alternatives.

Apart from the later radical interpretations of Freud, noted below, the social scientific survey work of Alfred Kinsey *et al.*(23) led to incontestable conclusions which helped establish the case of liberal/libertarian sex education. For Kinsey's massive questionnaire surveys disturbed the statistical pillar of sexual normality by discovering within the United States, great intra-cultural variation in sexual behaviour, identifying heterosexual intercourse as only one of six forms of sexual outlet (including: masturbation, nocturnal emission, heterosexual petting, homosexual relations and bestiality). His conclusions challenged assumptions about the nature of 'deviancy' and the validity of bio-sexual identities; for example, that there exists the genus 'homosexual' rather than men who (may) express a range of homosexual tendencies. Researches from a variety of disciplines continue to pursue answers to the question whether there is a scientific concept of normality which homosexuality violates.(24) Few other subjects within the field of sex education cause so much anxiety, making the subject the test case of all sex education. Scientific theorising and evidence will continue to play a vital political role in how this subject is dealt with at all levels of society (see below).

Social anthropology, sociology and the heritage of Kinsey's original surveys of sexual behaviour established that sexuality is contingent upon the culture in which it is expressed, and therefore displays variations. Weeks has made the point that this work provided a critical standard by which we began to judge the historical nature of our own societies, quoting the example of the influence Margaret Mead's 'Coming of Age in Samoa' had on 1930s American psychology by demonstrating that the (repressive) American way of dealing with adolescent 'deviance' was neither desirable, inevitable or necessary.(25)

Critical Social Science and Sexology

The tradition of 'critical theory', represented for much of this century in the work of the Frankfurt School of Sociology devoted much attention to the relationship between sexuality and society. For example, the Freudo-Marxism, represented in the post-war works of Wilhelm Reich and 1960s' theories of Herbert Marcuse, developed the notion that the liberation of sexual desire constituted a precondition of political freedom and an end to class oppression (with the corollary that sexual repression has underlying political causes). (26) Where such political analyses of sexuality have had any influence on the thinking of sex educators it is more likely to have been in the form of teachers' identification with the general spirit of sexual liberalisation during the 1960s and 1970s, when the writings of these authors were in vogue, rather than through any serious application of their work to the subject of sex education. This spirit was encapsulated in the Danish political self-help guide for the young: 'The Little Red School Book', which contained passages recommending sexual self-determination for the young which scandalised sections of British society in the early 1970s.(27) .

However, the subsequent application of critical social theory to the field of sexology has produced a vast output, particularly in the form of feminist critique, the influence of which on society is wide-ranging and long-lasting. Of the modern sexological sciences, Weeks comments:

'Over the past decade or so much has changed...There has been a minor explosion of historical writings about sex. We now know a great deal about such topics as marriage and the family, prostitution and homosexuality, the forms of legal and medical regulation, pre-Christian and non-Christian moral codes, women's bodies and health, illegitimacy and birth control, rape and sexual violence, the evolution of sexual identities and the importance of social networks and oppositional sexualities...Historians have deployed sophisticated methods of family reconstitution and demographic history... The history of sexuality may not yet be a respectable field of enquiry... but it now has a degree of professional recognition...'(28)

Applied to the phenomenon of human sexuality, critical social theory has embarked on the path of 'de-construction' of its historical components. Weeks acknowledges a debt to Foucault in inaugurating this process. The latter has contributed a history of the 'idea' of sexuality, itself, to the investigation of the causes and forms of sexual behaviour. In contrast to the conventional perception of sexuality as a natural phenomenon, Foucault perceived sexuality as 'a relationship of elements, a series of meaning-giving practices and activities, a social apparatus which had a history.'(29) This being so, sexuality may then be subjected to a critical analysis, which Weeks perceives as having three dimensions. The third dimension has profound implications for any sex education which purports to justify itself on scientific as well as merely desired moral principles:

'Firstly,... How is sexuality shaped; how is it articulated with economic, social and political structures, in a phrase, how is it socially constructed? Second, how and why has the domain of sexuality achieved such a critical organising and symbolic significance in Western culture; why do we think it is so important? Third: what is the relationship between sex and power; what role should we assign class divisions, pattern of male domination and racism? Coursing through each of these questions is a recurrent preoccupation: if sexuality is constructed by human agency, to what extent can it be changed?'(30)

Offering an alternative theoretical framework with which to address the phenomenon of sexual diversity uncovered by Kinsey, critical social theory has challenged the assumed 'naturalness' of the dominant sex roles, the 'normality' of heterosexual monogamy, and the notion of an invisible biological imperative of reproduction of the species expressed in sexual intercourse. From this perspective, human physiology is regarded as merely providing a set of physical possibilities for sexual relations, rather than determining what these relations must be.

Sexuality perceived as in large part a social construction has led to an appreciation of the relationship between sex, class and power: in particular, female subordination. Feminist critical perspectives were directed in the first instance at societies and social relations; the nuclear family, in particular, has been singled out as the principal means of female economic oppression, denial of female sexuality and sexual choice, and a vehicle for the transmission of capitalist society. Necessarily, this critique has been turned upon the historical construction of scientific sexology, itself. Consequently, sexual knowledge is exposed as defining sexuality in masculine terms, reflecting the (conscious and unconscious) interests of the dominant (male) scientific disciplines:

> '...feminists have argued that, "The ideology of sexuality has a material basis, and its basis is of course the division between men and women as this is organised through the monogamous patriarchal family". Their aim has been to examine how knowledge about sexuality has been organised to perpetuate this arrangement. Consequently, feminists have had, "to contend with some powerful myths", most notably the belief that "sex is a purely natural phenomenon and therefore apolitical", that its natural form of expression is heterosexuality, and that a woman's own sense of her sexuality is natural rather than socially constructed.'(31)

Moving beyond the now familiar critique of 'classical' Freudian psychoanalysis (phallocentric bias), feminists have also returned to the psychoanalytic tradition with new interpretations, with the objective of answering certain persistent sexological problems. In particular, there remains the need to explain why sexual identities *feel* so compelling even though the de-constructionist anthropological and sociological approaches suggest that these identities are in fact contingent, socially organised and even changeable.

Psychoanalytic theory reinterpreted can also be used to challenge the rigid distinctions made between men and women and the centrality of reproduction. The unconscious is seen to have its own dynamic, rules and history - a sphere of conflict of ideas, wishes and (sexual) desires, denied access to conscious life by the force of mental repression. This understanding of the workings of the unconscious proposes that individuals are not predetermined biological products; rather that their sexual identity as male, female, hetero- or homosexual, is a consequence of a psychic (Oedipal) conflict as the sexually polymorphous infant progresses through the stages of sexual development. This is described as an 'epic struggle', the outcome of which is uncertain:

> 'There is no inevitable progress to the altar of proper behaviour. If the process "worked" automatically there would be no ambiguity

about gender, no homosexuality, fetishism, transvestism and so on.'(32)

Injecting cultural significance into the Oedipal conflict provides an explanation of, 'how sexed identities are shaped in a complex human process through which anatomical differences acquire meaning in unconscious life'....'Our destinies are shaped not so much by the (anatomical) differences themselves but by their meaning, which is socially given and psychically elaborated.' Consequently, '(sexual) identities...are subject to disruptions all the time, through the eruption of unconscious elements, repressed desires...' Anatomy merely predisposes the individual toward sexual identity rather than determines this identity: 'pre-existing structures of sexual difference... limit the free play of desire and the pursuit of other differences, other ways of being human.'(33)

Sexuality, then, is to be explained in terms of a combination of *psychic structuring* and the (conscious) *acquisition of pre-existing social forms*. The latter component has been elaborated by reference to the learning of sexual 'scripts'. Reiss has defined sexual scripts in the following way:

> 'I use the term cultural script to mean a shared group definition of the type of situation, type of people and type of behaviour appropriate in a particular social context. There are cultural scripts aimed at producing an erotic response in the participants, and I shall call these sexual scripts. The sexual scripts derive from the shared, consensual beliefs people have about what is good and bad sexuality in their society. These sexual scripts act as guides regarding what that society believes are the proper circumstances for experiencing an erotic response.... Some degree of change is inevitable for the shared sexual scripts cannot possibly spell out every action, thought and feeling that should occur. In this sense the individual is constantly "editing" the sexual scripts of his or her society.'(34)

Recent history provides spectacular examples of the ways in which sexual scripts have been *socially* created, modified, and adopted, uniting those with common 'psychic' dispositions. Ironically, the pursuit of measures of sexual normality by the positive sciences have played a hand in this by creating sexual identities through the technique of classification. The 19th century sexologists chose to classify observed behaviours according to 'deviations' from the 'normal'. Kinsey preferred the more scientifically- neutral classification of sexual 'diversity'. Either way, this process interfered with the objects of sexology by presenting the public with a range of sexual scripts out of which new identities could be acquired to suit psychic dispositions. As science isolated the homosexual 'identity' in the 19th century, providing a sexual script for the creation of a distinct sexual subculture, so political changes have permitted such subcultures a public voice:

> 'As the homosexual ways of life have become more public and self-confident, so in their wake other assertions of minority sexual identities have emerged. The example of homosexuality, as Gayle Rubin, has argued, has provided a repertoire of political strategies and organisational forms for the mobilisation of other erotic populations. Transvestites, transsexuals, paedophiles, sado-masochists, fetishists, bisexuals, prostitutes and others have vocally emerged, clamouring for their right to self expression and legitimacy....These new sexual and social identities may have emerged on the terrain first mapped and carefully articulated by the sexologists, themselves.' (35)

The Implications of 'Critical Sexology' for Sex Education

The emergence of a science of sexuality over the last two centuries has resulted in the development of competing theories of sexual orientation and behaviour. It is fair to say that during this period there has been progress made in understanding how sexual identity and behaviour is actively acquired rather than inherited as a form of instinctual behaviour, though disagreements remain over how this 'learning' occurs.

More importantly, the application of critical social theory to the history of sexology has revealed how conventional scientific methods have served an ideological purpose under the guise of objectivity. As sexological facts have fallen under the scrutiny of an alternative scientific method, so has the sex education which had been erected on these facts. Thus, those concerned with the way in which female sexuality has been described, charge that ideology has everywhere been disguised as fact; that sex education has incorporated a masculine view of sexuality defined in reproductive terms in which the male is seen as active and dominant and the female as passive and receptive:

> 'Sex education's common reduction of sexuality to reproduction not only equates sex to intercourse, but also is not concerned with young people's present experience, preferring to prepare them for future defined roles'...'Girls are extremely unlikely to learn about the nature of their own sexual response from the vast majority of sex education books...when there is a political drive towards reproduction, aimed at economic or social reorganisation, then this denial of women's sexuality has an ideological purpose, as equally does the assertion of male dominance, which consists of the maintenance of male gender roles, which are additionally reinforced

through sex education's deliberate omission of male and female homosexuality.'... 'This kind of attitude does not help or ease the anxiety felt by many adolescents about their sexual identity, or promote understanding of the depth and breadth of human sexual feelings...' (36)

The scientific perception of sexuality as a 'learning' process (however complex), rather than as a biological conditioning, through which changes in orientation might be possible through self-reflection, de-stabilises the moral code which the latter provide for. The comfortable division between sexual normality and deviancy/perversity is undermined by a recognition of sexual 'diversity'. Moreover, the ethics of tolerance of (and even 'treatment' for) fixed sexual endowments are no longer relevant if such behaviours can potentially be acquired, enjoyed, defended or even unlearned.

It is necessary to conclude that, in the pursuit of 'truth', successive sexologies have discredited and replaced previously-established facts. In so doing, what passed as a scientific underpinning of certain traditional values has been removed. All of this represents a serious threat to defenders of traditional sexual ethics, roles and education. For they are forced either to dispute the scientific basis of the feminist critique and the evidence it has brought to bear, or instead to expound an alternative non-scientific legitimacy for their preferred sexual value-system, such as Christianity.

Traditionalists will be forced to dispute not merely the 'facts' feminists have established but their whole scientific approach, because critical theory is built upon a scientific paradigm wedded to liberation rather than control. The division made by Habermas between the 'natural sciences' and the 'sciences of social action', if sound, reveals the connection between the scientific method, its object and the rationale it carries with it:

'In the empirical-analytic sciences the frame of reference that prejudges the meaning of possible statements establishes rules both for the construction of theories and for their critical testing. Theories comprise hypothetico-deductive connections of propositions which permit the deduction of lawlike hypotheses with empirical content....The systematic sciences of social action, that is economics, sociology and political science, have the goal as do the empirical-analytic sciences of producing nomological knowledge. A critical social science, however, will not remain satisfied with this. It is concerned with going beyond this goal to determine when theoretical statements grasp invariant regularities of social action as such and when they express ideologically frozen relations of dependence that can in principle be transformed. To the extent that this is the case, the critique of ideology, as well moreover, as psychoanalysis, takes into account that information about lawlike connections sets off a process of reflection in the consciousness of those the laws are about... (self-reflection)... releases the subject from dependence on hypostatised powers. Self-reflection is determined by an emancipatory cognitive interest.'(37)

If sexuality is in the final analysis more a social phenomenon than a determinate biological one, it must be subject to the corresponding scientific paradigm and the rationale derived from it.

A relatively 'unproblematic' socio-political management of sexuality had been guaranteed by the scientific sexology organised according to the 'natural science' paradigm. Thus, positive sexology helped reaffirm the moral superiority of (statistically) 'normal' monogamous, heterosexual, adult, genital/reproductive sexual behaviour by its organisation of knowledge. Deviations could be classified and explained causally by reference to whatever determining factors which happened to be the focus of the discipline: biology, chemicals, genes, animal heredity, and so on. Changes in sexual behaviour might be more or less possible according to adjustment of objective conditions - tampering with 'nature'. Equally unproblematic has been the moral education which has been erected around these sciences, insofar as such education is more or less exclusively concerned with 'control'(the 'medical model'). That is, social control of what is sexually possible, and sexual self-control.

By contrast, the 'emancipatory' impetus of the 'critical sexologies' has had a powerful impact both on many progressive teachers, and their traditionalist critics. Some of the former now recognise that their sex education role is one which is dedicated to freeing their pupils as early in their lives as possible from what are seen as socially and personally destructive sex roles. Meanwhile the latter complain of the mass of conflicting ideas and ideologies imported into the classroom, and the 'amoralism' which some teachers promote by encouraging sexual self-determination.

Modes of teaching have evolved to accompany this shift in perception of sexuality, though the historico-political process appears to be approaching a full circle, as the following diagram displays, derived from the work of Bernstein and Douglas(38).

The shift from Cell A to Cell B has been addressed above. Cell C describes the emergence of the 'experiential', child-centred progressivism which characterised much of British pedagogical thinking in the 1970s. In the 1980s,

FIG 1

GRID REPRESENTING MODES OF SEX EDUCATION TEACHING (39)

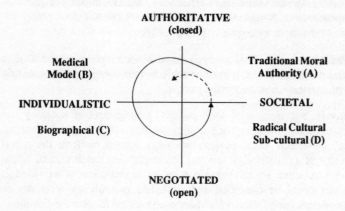

this approach applied to sex education is only one of many educational fields in which it is under attack.

There are two issues raised by this current crisis: firstly, there is a danger that both defenders and detractors of recent sexological theories misrepresent what these theories are proposing, for the sake of their wider moral or political interests. For example, an over-simplistic conception of sexual 'script'-learning has appeared in the form of a pervasive anxiety that exposure to information about homosexuality during adolescence, which challenges the 'abnormality' label traditionally applied to it, may engender a 'drift' towards this sexual orientation by some young people, which would not otherwise occur. This is hardly the kind of learning process sexologists have in mind when they state that sexual orientation may become 'fixed' through early psychic processes, than through a natural disposition.(40)

Secondly, there is a danger that the value basis of 'critical sexology' and its rationale become regarded as synonymous with school sex education. While sex education must draw upon the findings and argumentation of critical sexology, neither the classroom nor the teacher-pupil relationship are suitable vehicles to take a radical or dominant role in sexual socialisation by subjecting facts and values to full-scale critique. It is the task of the school to assist in the process of enabling the young person to understand and where necessary to survive society's conflicting signals, to recognise and absorb its higher values, and to value its more durable structures (eg. the family). This involves as much a process of individual *accommodation* to the sexual status quo, as acquiring the means to discriminate the negative and positive elements of it.

With this separation of function established, all sides of the political spectrum have much to gain from the critique of sexual determinism. For it is arguable that a scientific theorising which locates, for example, male sexual aggression in 'complex social practices and psychic structuring'(41) holds out a better prospect for humane relations between the sexes than one which must reconcile the young to innate gender 'drives'. If sex roles and behaviour are, in the final analysis a matter of such drives, sex education must remain founded upon a rationale of control over instincts and geared to protection of the sexes from the permanent threat posed by each to the other. If the former, such education holds out the possibility of discriminating between negative and positive learned expressions of masculinity and femininity in accord with the higher values to which society adheres.

Scientific inquiry, cannot be regarded as a 'neutral' procedure, but carries with it its own constituting rationale. The moral guidelines which are to be the 'end-product' of sex education will emerge from the social theories of which the knowledge base is comprised; they cannot be decided independently of this knowledge base or imposed on it (even though this is what some interest groups might wish).

The current clamour for the teaching of more 'facts' and less politics is redundant insofar as the 'objective' status of knowledge about human sexuality now depends upon whether those concerned with it are willing to concede the shift in scientific paradigm, and the implications this has for past and present sexological theory and data described above. The alternative is to countenance only that knowledge which supports preferred sex roles and relations - which is no scientific basis at all, or to ignore criteria of a scientific nature in favour of a purely moral standpoint.

Notes

1. *Parliamentary Debates* House of Lords Official Report Vol 367 No 18 14th January 1976 HMSO col 136

2. see the media coverage of Clause 28 of the 1988 Local Government Bill concerning homosexuality.

3. see the arguments contained in the publications of the Responsible Society; for example Rogers, A 'Sex Lessons' *Times Health Supplement* February 5th 1982

4. see Introduction, chapter 1 above.

5. Clarity Collective *Taught Not Caught* , Cousins, *Make it Happy* Virago 1978

6. Allen I *Education in Sex and Personal Relationships* Policy Studies Institute, London pg 184

7. *Parliamentary Debates* House of Lords 1976 op cit. col 142.

8. Weeks, J *Sex, Politics and Society: The Regulation of Sexuality Since 1800* Longman, Harlow 1981; *Sexuality and Its Discontents: Meanings, Myths and Modern Sexualities* Routledge Kegan Paul, London 1985; *Sexuality* Ellis Horwood/ Tavistock Publications, London 1986

9. Wallis, G P *Some Ideological Issues in Sex Education in Post-War Britain* unpublished MA Dissertation. University of London Institute of Education September 1984

10. Weeks, J 1986 op cit. pg 13

11. *Parliamentary Debates* House of Lords 1976 op cit. col 160ff

12. Weeks, J 1986 op cit. pg 14

13. Wallis, G 1984 op cit. pg 48

14. Newsom, J *The Education of Girls* Faber & Faber 1948 pg 109

15. ibid. pg 12

16. Newsom, J *Central Advisory Council for Education* pg 54

17. see Reiff, P *The Triumph of the Therapeutic* Penguin, Harmondsworth 1966; Halmos, P *The Faith of the Counsellors* Constable, London 1965; Heraud, B J *Sociology and Social Work: Perspectives and Problems* Pergamon Press, Oxford 1970

18. quoted in Wallis, G 1984 op cit. pg 68

19. ibid. quoting Corner: *Attaining manhood: A Doctor talks to Boys about Sex* Harper and Bros. 1938; Richards, L *For Boys* Basil Blackwell, Oxford 1963; Picton, M *Understanding Parenthood and Childcare* Blackie 1980

20. Weeks, J 1985 op cit pg 113-4

21. quoted in Wallis, G 1984 op cit pg 35

22. Reiss, I L. *Journey Into Sexuality* Prentice-Hall, Englewood Cliffs, New Jersey 1986 pg 4; see also Archer, J and Lloyd, B *Sex and Gender* Penguin Harmondsworth 1982

23. Kinsey, A *et al. Sexual Behaviour in the Human Male* Saunders, Philadelphia 1948; *Sexual Behaviour in the Human Female* Saunders, Philadelphia 1953

24. see Reiss, I L 1986 op cit.

25. Weeks, J 1986 op cit pg 22

26. for a review of the influence of these authors see: Robinson, P A *The Sexual Radicals: Reich, Roheim, Marcuse* Paladin, London 1972.

27. Hansen, S and Jensen, J *The Little Red Schoolbook* Stage 1 (English Translation 1971). This text was the subject of a legal prohibition by the Department of Public Prosecutions under the Obscene Publications Act. The publisher, R Handyside took the case unsuccessfully to the European Court of Human Rights.

28. Weeks, J 1986 op cit. pg 19-20

29. ibid. pg 23

30. ibid. pg 23

31. Wallis, G 1984 op cit. pg 92, quoting McIntosh, M in Women's Study Group (eds) *Women Take Issue: Aspects of Women's Subordination* Centre for Contemporary Cultural Studies, Hutchinson Birmingham 1978 pg 63; Coote, A and Campbell, B *Sweet Freedom: The Struggle for Women's Liberation* Picador 1982 pg 212

32. Weeks, J 1986 op cit. pg 62

33. ibid. pg 64

34. Reiss, I L op cit. pg 20-25

35. Weeks, J 1986 op cit. pg 77

36. Wallis, G 1984 op cit. pg 94

37. Habermas, J *Knowledge and Human Interests* Heinemann London 1978 pg 309-310

38. Bernstein, B *Class, Codes and Control* Vol 1, *Theoretical Studies Towards a Sociology of Language,* London, Routledge Kegan Paul 1977; Douglas, M *Natural Symbols*, Pelican, Penguin, Harmondsworth 1973

39. This representation was developed by Alan Beattie as part of the IPPF Europe Project on European Sex Education Trends; Report Forthcoming

40. see Mitchell, J *Psychoanalysis and Feminism* Allen Lane, London 1974

41. Weeks, J 1986 op cit. pg 65

Chapter 4

Psychological Roots of 'Traditionalism' and 'Progressivism'

This study looks primarily to political explanations to the question why is it so difficult to acquire the social consensus necessary to organise a rational programme of sex education in schools. Religio-cultural heritage provides one powerful source of resistance to any attempt to change a society's traditional approach to aspects of social behaviour surrounded with moral injunction. Such 'ideological' resistance materialises in forms of campaigning of a political kind; the stimulation of mass opinion in favour of one set of arguments against another by competing interest groups. Resistance to such change also appears indirectly through the workings of bureaucracies whose responsibility it is to manage the educational process. Such bureaucracies operate according to rules of self-maintenance and protection from superior powers rather than simply according to their explicit function of implementing decisions, legislation or regulations from above. At the end of the day, bureaucracies are made up of individual decision-makers whose rule-following will depend upon personal as well as extraneous organisational interests.

In modern societies there are many differences of opinion over means and ends of sex education which must be resolved 'rationally'. This may take the form of appeal to: authority, the democratic process, persuasion, appeal to scientific proof, and so on. However, in addition, it is likely that decision-making on issues of sex education is exceptional in the degree to which any number of rational compromises are inhibited by powerful motives. This is to propose that the politics of sex education has a psychological dimension on which it is only possible to speculate, but which should be recognised in any comprehensive explanation of this social reality.

There are undeniably powerful emotional reasons for the strength of argument of many individuals with a vested interest in the development of the subject in schools. Where traditionally-minded politicians capitalise upon (latent) public resistance to Governmental moves to direct sex education in one way or another, some may be out merely to capitalise upon the opportunity to turn public opinion against the political opponent. However, in this field it is clear that most also express rather unarticulated but nevertheless deeply-felt concerns of a more emotional kind. The same applies to those spokespersons

62

of moral movements who attribute immoral and anti-social intent to sex education reformers.

Many objections to organised sex education as a means of 'enlightening' the young are easy to sympathise with, without recourse to psychology. One of these is the demand that it is the sole right of parents rather than public officials to educate about morality. Others include that such knowledge, given at too young an age, will corrupt or lead to irresponsible behaviour by the immature. It is also felt that to 'objectify' sexuality in the form of a public education inevitably de-bases what may be felt to be a deeply private and even sacred part of life. There is much concern about the health risks of sexual behaviour at a young age, and that to learn is to practice. Recently in Britain, it has been argued that certain teachers cannot be trusted to provide what parents believe are the correct values. Alternatively, defenders of 'enlightening' sex education draw upon motives which stem from a wish to remove the ignorance and anxieties for this subject which they experienced when young.

Both critics and defenders are likely to be reacting in part to past or present anxieties about their own sexuality. One may even go so far as to say that beliefs are protecting individuals against anxieties arising from hidden problems which to some extent remain unresolved. Such is the human condition. Weeks has summarised this situation thus:

> 'Despite sustained attempts over many years to "demystify" sex, and several decades of much proclaimed- or condemned- "liberalism" and "permissiveness", the erotic still arouses acute moral anxiety and confusion. This is not because sex is intrinsically "naughty", as a sensitive commentator has rightly remarked, "but because it is a focus for powerful feelings". The strong emotions it undoubtedly arouses give to the world of sexuality a seismic sensitivity making it a transmission belt for a wide variety of needs and desires: for love and anger, tenderness and aggression, intimacy and adventure, romance and predatoriness, pleasure and pain, empathy and power.'
> (1)

Sex education is perceived as one means of learning to understand and 'manage' anxiety-creating 'animal drives' in human beings. However, in order to do this it must bring them into conscious reflection. This is the first source of anxiety for many. A society's culture is an adaptive mechanism, not only to the outer but inner (psychic) world. It may be understood as a system of defence mechanisms against anxieties about the individual self. This may be seen in the way a society decides upon what are permissible and not permissible conceptualisations and displays of sexuality.

Sex education generates powerful emotions which influence the way conscious decision-making takes place. Sexuality itself produces anxieties at an individual level. It is well known that the 'objectification' of sexuality in order that it be susceptible to rational reflection and management for educational purposes is hindered by problems of legitimate and illegitimate vocabularies - socially acceptable/ meaningful versus socially unacceptable/ meaningless ways of articulating bodily parts, actions, feelings and relationships according to audience.

In *The Ostrich Position*, Carol Lee has described her experiences of educationalists who have strongly objected to what in contemporary society should be uncontentious sex education material. In one example she quotes a health education panel objecting to the use of the word 'vagina' being used in a film being made about menstruation. One member physician forcefully objected to this though he was unable to explain why he felt 'uncomfortable' with it. She concludes:

> '...people who are designated decision-makers and who hold the power of deciding how young people are to receive information, are in such a state of basic confusion that they perpetuate attitudes they do not believe they hold. They are, in other words, deluded. If challenged they would be outraged to be told that they were obstructing the course of education.' (2)

Weeks has recalled sociologist Ken Plummer's comment that sex research still makes you 'morally suspect'. (3) So much the more so those individuals and movements which have set out to provide a form of education about sexuality for young people as a means of sparing them unnecessary anxieties and ignorance. But this should be an expected reaction to those who propose to remove defence-mechanisms through 'public' education.

How might this anxiety about the young gaining 'public' access to what is a taboo area of adult consciousness be explained. In examining 20 indices of sexuality across 186 non-industrial cultures, Reiss provides some clues in his identification of two key universal characteristics of sexuality: 'self-disclosure' and 'physical pleasure' (the cultural labelling of body parts as erotic). By self-disclosure, he refers to the making known to another some previously unknown aspect of oneself. Self-disclosure affords the other person a deeper understanding of what one is like. The more complete the disclosure, the more intimate and private are the things being shown. Sexual self-disclosure also reveals *vulnerability* (need for tenderness/ affection) and child-like qualities of adults (for comfort etc) which clash strongly particularly with the male role in everyday life.

Self-disclosure provides one clue to the strength of anxiety about 'public' sex education and the access to human feeling which sexual knowledge bestows. For much adult experience of sexual life - the self-disclosing process - is likely to have been far from perfect; in fact a source of pain as much as pleasure. Where the emotional experience of sexuality has been unhappy it is more likely to be buried from consciousness as a form of self-protection. Sex education exposes the subject to discussion, bringing it into a process of reflection the limits to which, for adults, are unclear and left to the imagination. This can foster anxiety which expresses itself in defence of the pupil. 'Public' (school) sex education provides the child with a means of mental access to the private existence of the parent, delivered by an outsider. If the family is a closed psychological unit, sex education allows an outsider into one highly charged dimension of it through the child.

Physical pleasure offers the means of a second speculation on the source of motives for resistance to organised sexual learning. The physical and interpersonal rewards which sexual relations can offer can be short lived and are not easy to obtain by every adult in a relationship. In fact, lack or loss of sexual fulfilment is the fate of many (Reiss reminds us of the large number of anorgasmic women in conventional marriages). It is arguable that prurient antagonism to adolescents' pursuit of sexual knowledge (both intellectually and physically), however rationalised, concealed an envy for the kind of physical and emotional fulfilment which is now a publicly-displayed part of this time of life.

Sections of the media are renowned for exploiting the voyeuristic anxieties of their adult readership in delivering them real or imaginary examples of the sexual behaviour of the young, free of the social constraints to which adult society is resigned to conform. Like the culture hero in traditional religious movements, the media (and moral campaigners) act as a mouthpiece of the sum of the unconscious wishes of the other individuals in the society. Reflecting upon this, the Swedish National Board of Education discussion of the rationale for sex education felt it necessary to state:

'Contrary to what some people imagine, the main purpose of regular association during the teens is not that of arranging "sheer" sexual gratification without any personal regard for the opposite number. In most cases it is unfair to young persons to make such an allegation.' (4)

In his study of the cultural 'universals' of sexuality, Reiss identifies 'jealousy' as a boundary-setting mechanism for what the group feels are important relationships; defining the legitimate boundaries of important relationships such as marriage. When these normative boundaries are violated, jealousy occurs. In their first sexual encounter/s young people operate outside the normative boundaries (marriage) to which adult society is expected to, but does not always, conform. Marriage is the most valued home of the sexual relationship. This union of sexuality and marriage is what marital sexual jealousy is protecting. (5)

Sex education is concerned in part with the ground rules for sexual relationships; in this respect it offers measures of 'ideal' possible relations. In practice, few sexual relationships conform with this ideal, but are rather a focus for occasional doubt, anxiety, even guilt. The fear of sex education is the fear of exposure of the real versus the ideal ground rules of sexual relations which are so tenuous in many adult lives. One way of reducing the possibility of this exposure is to control the direction of this education such as by removing it from the classroom and returning it to the family.

It remains to describe how these anxieties are expressed in the form of politics.

Notes

1. Weeks, J *Sexuality* Tavistock 1986 pg 11

2. Lee C *The Ostrich Position* Readers and Writers, London pg 8

3. Plummer, K *Sexual Stigma: An Interactionist Account* Routledge & Kegan Paul London 1975 pg 4

4. Swedish National Board of Education *Instruction Concerning Interpersonal Relations* 1981 Liber Stockholm 1981

5. Reiss, J *Journey into Sexuality* Academic Press, Englewood Cliffs, New Jersey 1987 pg 56

Chapter 5

The Political Management of School Sex Education in England

It has been argued above that an increase in the provision of school sex education and its dissemination throughout the curriculum has been achieved often through schools shielding themselves from controversy, by ensuring that the content and style of teaching remain relatively closed to public scrutiny. It is a credit to teachers and head teachers who have designed or adopted programmes and carried out such teaching in the knowledge that they may be exposed to criticism from the partisan positions of national and local media, political groups and parents. However, the price paid for this secrecy, nationally, is a climate of political doubt and mistrust fed by media exposes of 'unacceptable' teaching. This contrasts with actual evidence of any wane in the confidence of the 'public' in the role played by the teaching profession in offering factual knowledge within a moral framework acceptable to the majority.

Parliament has, over the past 10 years, begun to challenge this status quo by means of a series of legal amendments which affect the power structures within which sex education is taught, some of which have failed to gain consensus necessary to become law and others which have succeeded.

It is recognised that there is little likelihood that differences in attitudes to moral and sexual issues can be eliminated in the foreseeable future. However, the political momentum towards new forms of teacher 'accountability', standardisation and standard setting in the school curriculum demands that at some time in the future this subject be scrutinised rationally in order that it be established as an approved component of the whole national curriculum. It was argued in previous chapters that a *sine qua non* of this process is some form of review and systematic organisation of and approach to selecting from the knowledge base of the subject.

It is proposed here that future comprehensive curriculum guidelines are only likely to be integrated into, and bear fruit in, the educational system if they become indispensable to the operation of the relevant part of that system. To discover how this might be so requires a *strategic* explanation of the political-administrative structure relevant to sex education. That is to say, an elucidation of how *power* is manifested and used. For this structure decides

67

how sex education is to be defined, how, or whether, it is to be provided at all. Improvements in the content and teaching of sex education have depended, and will continue to depend, upon access to power in the structure, though power in this case is subtle and elusive.

Most competing interest-groups which have a stake in the development of school sex education have attempted in one way or another to manipulate the political structure with which this field is governed, through the appeal of their ideologies. Supporters and sympathisers are recruited from Parliament and the professions in order to gain a voice in the decision-making process affecting school education. While the 'political' issue of sex education is well known from the point of view of the ideologies of its protagonists, it is less understood how the political structure has affected the development of sex education through the allocation of power to one sector rather than another.

For political purposes beyond the advancement of sex education in schools, the present government has already undertaken its own strategic review of this structure, leading to legislative and regulatory measures designed to shift power over the curriculum.

The Political Management of Sex Education: A Theory of Power

It is not obvious how 'power' is manifested in the politico-bureaucratic management of sex education, though it is possible as in any political process to recognise examples of its various forms: authority, influence, manipulation and coercion. This is partly because of the intangibility and hidden nature of the subject, often revealed as little more than a negotiation of ideas or 'desiderata', rather than the organisation of a substantive curriculum. Interest groups have competed with one another over definitions of the subject, and the prime locus of power - government - has intervened when controversy of the subject has posed a threat to its wider interests, as much as out of a genuine concern to assist in its development and implementation.

Moreover, sex education is an uncertain means to attaining uncertain ends. There might be wide consensus over the need to encourage morally/sexually responsible adolescent behaviour through such education, but less agreement over how much, and what kind of, knowledge is necessary to achieve this. It is also a matter of some anguish whether the full sense of the word 'education' should really apply to this field in these years - in its sense of enlightenment and the nurturing of an analytic and critical faculty.

As a result of these imponderables, in this area of education, apart perhaps from the earliest post war years, the management process has rarely taken the simple form of the higher national power securing the commitment and compliance of the subordinate regional and semi-dependent authorities to work towards an agreed objective. Such are the sensitivities generated by the subject that it has been more the case that virtually every authority in the process has resorted to some bureaucratic means or another to ensure that their own 'stake' in the subject, or interests relating to it, remain paramount. This applies equally to the independent, semi-independent and higher governmental authorities.

Although government is the prime legislative body regarding initiatives in the development of school sex education, it is not usually the best qualified to decide what form this development should take. Hence, the task is often 'sub-contracted' to semi- and fully independent bodies which are believed to possess some expertise in this field. However, where a subject of education lacks an orthodoxy to the extent that sex education does, this delegation of responsibility carries certain risks. All political decision-making involves the risk of criticism from competing interest groups. However, such criticism is based upon pragmatic or policy considerations. In the case of sex education, there exists an added basis for criticism based on a questioning of motives relating to sexual morality.

Those organisations involved in managing sex education as a bureaucratic responsibility appear to be as vulnerable to this threat as campaigning organisations with an investment in the promotion of the subject in one form or another. This added dimension (perhaps unique within education) is referred to here as the threat of moral discredit. *Moral discredit* might be conceived as a potential side-effect of any attempt to confront or otherwise manipulate the subject. It has a powerful effect upon the way sex education is managed throughout the politico-educational system. Government is as susceptible to 'contamination' with moral discredit as any other interest-group in the structure, including at the other extreme, the teacher in the classroom.

It is argued here that, while the binding force of legislation might be regarded as the most concrete manifestation of power in matters of sex education, strategic use of 'threat of exposure to moral discredit' (from which follows political discredit) has been far more pervasive and influential. All actors in the structure, including parliamentary government, must protect themselves from moral discredit by others. The fear of moral discredit has given vocal individuals in Parliament the power to influence the funding for whole organisations (as in the early 1980s case of Catholic MP James Pawsey versus Brook Advisory Centres).(1) Alternatively moral discredit is a valuable weapon in a form of party political 'smear campaigns'. There is an element of this in the current Conservative-proposed amendment to the 1988 Local Government Bill, Clause 28 of which proposes to forbid any 'promotion' of homosexuality in schools or in any other activity funded by local authorities. In this case, the existence of left-wing gay political groups was used to embarrass Labour Party-controlled local authorities, which have chosen to defend the rights of such groups (the so-called 'looney left' is now an established (and influential) 'folk devil' of the conservative media and certain Conservative politicians).

In each case the individual or body threatening moral discredit challenges those who would question the threat to defend themselves publicly. Few are willing to expose themselves in this way to 'contamination' by moral discredit in the sexual sphere for the political damage which may accrue.

The following proposes to show that parliamentarians and government ministries made use of or threatened to use moral discredit against governmental as well as non-governmental agencies whose activities in the sex education field have threatened its political power base. Where non-governmental organisations use ideology; and Parliamentarians and the press occasionally resort to scandal tactics; the government, itself, uses the legislature in the struggle both to survive moral discredit and at the same time secure its own popularity.

The politico-bureaucratic structure governing school sex education may be illustrated by means of the diagram on page 71.

The diagram displays the central government apparatus of policy-making through Parliament, where Ministers of Education and Health direct their Departments to create regulations. Using government-funded advisory bodies, such regulations may be given guidelines to assist civil service authorities integrate them into the curriculum, a process monitored by school inspectors or health education officers. The traditional autonomy of schools under the direction of the head teacher (reporting to the school governors) is limited by the obligation to conform with legislated guidelines regarding the school curriculum, though local autonomy will be exercised as to their interpretation. Teaching staff are expected to act in accord with the wishes of the head teacher, though this may be the result of collaboration. Traditionally, each school is answerable to a Local Education Authority (LEA), which in some cases attempts to influence head teachers through the production of policy papers and recommendations.

There are 163 LEAs in England and Wales, each responsible to central government and expected to promote national educational policies at the local level, as well as undertaking administrative functions. Thus, in theory, decision-making appears to be relatively hierarchical. In addition, the subject of sex education, in particular, has attracted a range of interest- or pressure-groups concerned to *influence* the creation and interpretation of regulations by official bodies. Each actor has something to gain and something

FIG 2.

POLITICAL AND ADMINISTRATIVE MANAGEMENT OF SCHOOL SEX EDUCATION IN ENGLAND

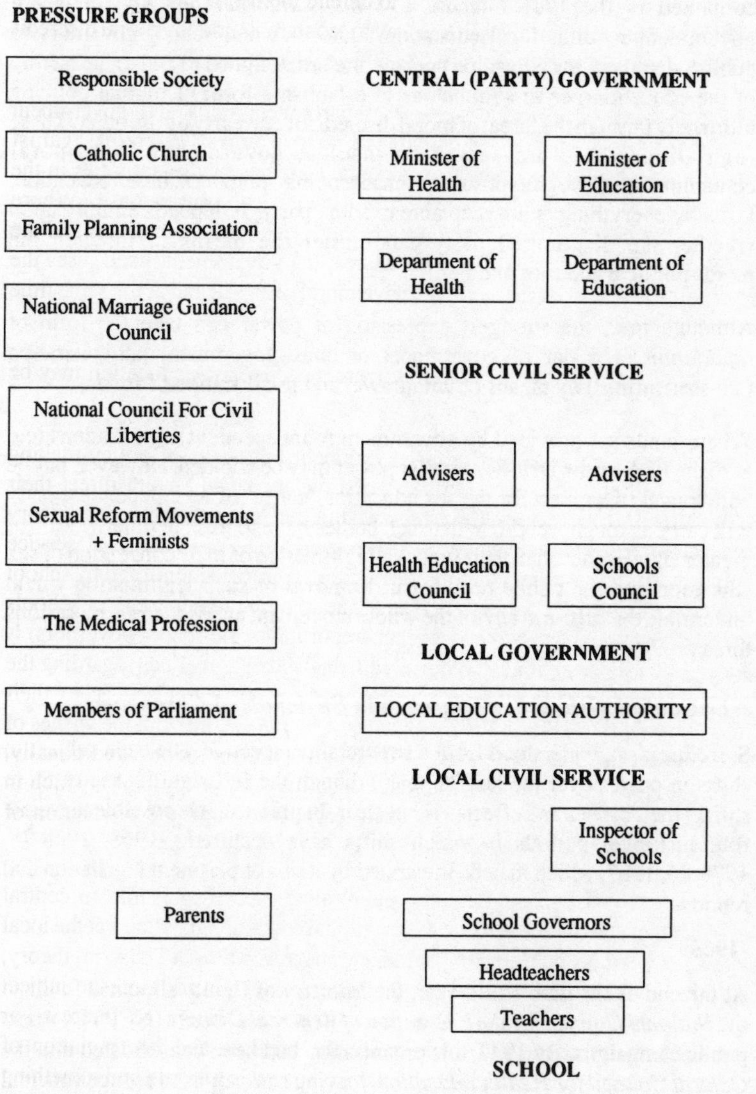

PRESSURE GROUPS

| Responsible Society |

CENTRAL (PARTY) GOVERNMENT

| Minister of Health | Minister of Education |

| Catholic Church |

| Department of Health | Department of Education |

| Family Planning Association |

| National Marriage Guidance Council |

SENIOR CIVIL SERVICE

| National Council For Civil Liberties |

| Advisers | Advisers |

| Sexual Reform Movements + Feminists |

| Health Education Council | Schools Council |

| The Medical Profession |

LOCAL GOVERNMENT

| Members of Parliament |

| LOCAL EDUCATION AUTHORITY |

LOCAL CIVIL SERVICE

| Inspector of Schools |

| Parents |

| School Governors |

| Headteachers |

| Teachers |

SCHOOL

to lose according to their preferred role in the structure. Within this particular power-structure it is rarely possible for one party to *force* (compliance by threat of deprivation) another party to act in a certain way, though options for action may be narrowed. It is more often the case that accountable subordinate authorities are prevented from acting in ways which might attract moral discredit to the higher authority. For this reason, regulations such as those contained in the 1981 *Education (Schools Information) Act,* in which government requires local education authorities and school governors to publish details of sex education courses, are not designed to add to the quality of the education per se so much as to establish a form of mutual policing ultimately through the threat of moral discredit of one party by the other. These regulations therefore served to insulate government from moral contamination through exposure of 'unacceptable' practices. In sex education, virtually everything is unacceptable to some party; it depends entirely upon whether the disgruntled party can muster the means to threaten the moral-political status of another.

Although rare, the strongest expression of power can take the form of *liquidation* of a tier of government or quasi-government administration ('re-structuring') by means of withdrawal and re-allocation of funds.

Where funds are provided by government to independent organisations (eg. as to the FPA by the DHSS) a similar power may be wielded. However, public withdrawal of support for the sex education 'cause' of an independent body will carry as much weight. What such bodies have to lose, in other words (of greater significance than their funds) is legitimation of *their* conception of sex education and the public need for it. Removal of such legitimation would undermine the *raison d' être* of the whole movement and is therefore a serious threat.

Who Controls School Sex Education in England?: A Chronology

Sex education, understood from a structural perspective, has been subject to shifts in power over the last 20 years, though the full significance of these shifts - their causes and effects - is not clear. In practice, it is possible to isolate four historical periods in which shifts have occurred: -1968, 1968-78, 1978-86, 1987, which may be illustrated by items of pertinent legislation and reports.

-1968

At the end of the first World War, the Ministry of Health allocated funds to the *National Council for the Prevention of Venereal Disease* (NCPVD) to run public campaigns. By 1927, this organisation had been consolidated into the *Central Council for Health Education,* leaving campaigns to reduce venereal diseases located alongside other public health campaigns. The first national, official codification of a nascent sex education came in 1928 with the Government *Board of Education's* 'Handbook of Suggestions on Health Education'. This publication offered an explicit moral code for schools and teachers, reinforcing the Victorian values of 'temperance, chastity and thrift'. This publication was to be re-published several times during the next 30 years.

The same year saw the publication of the *Hadow Report*: 'Education of the Adolescent', the first major government report on an educational topic. With its renewed emphasis on *sexual hygiene*, this report reaffirmed that any government interest in sexuality as a topic of education was confined solely to the containment of venereal disease. Henceforth it was recommended that teachers deal with this subject within domestic science and biology.

Towards the end of the Second World War, as part of its planned social reconstruction programme, a new legislative framework for state education was created which aimed to widen educational opportunity. This was to include sex education, even though the term remained implicit in the following directive (which was to remain until 1986):

'It should be the duty of the Local Education Authority for every area, so far as their powers extend, to contribute towards the spiritual, moral, mental and physical development of the community.'(2)

During the post war years this education contained a pronatalist message. Beveridge's report *Social Insurance and Allied Services* identified the family as the dominant social unit of reproduction:

'In the next thirty years housewives as mothers have vital work to do in ensuring the continuation of the British race and British ideals in the world.'(3)

The 1959 *Crowther Report* discussed changing social needs in relation to the education of this age group, noting that:

'It is surely gain that boys and girls, young men and women, should have the opportunity which earlier generations often lacked to get to know one another really well before committing themselves to the choice of a mate. It is surely a loss that new guiding rules of behaviour in the changed situation have not been sufficiently developed to replace the old customs which nearly everybody has to some extent abandoned and which some have altogether thrown overboard. Clearly it is not possible for an educational service which is designed to prepare the young for adult life, to establish by itself such a code. This is the concern of society as a whole, young and old alike. Education can only function within the broad directives of right and wrong which society gives. Teachers and youth leaders are, however, well placed to bring to attention the personal bewilderment and disaster to which this public indecision over moral issues often leads the young.'(4)

The 1963 *Newsom Report* 'Half Our Future', reviewed schooling for the 'less than average' pupil, assigning clear responsibility to schools for sex education, as revealed in the following passage:

'Positive guidance to boys and girls on sexual morals is essential, with quite specific discussion on the problems they will face. Advice to the parents on dealing with the problems of their children's physical and emotional adolescence may be equally needed, and should be easily available whether through the school or through the Health and Welfare Services.'

In looking at the sort of courses that should be provided, the Newsom report had this to say:

'One line of advance lies in the courses built around themes of home-making, to include not only material and practical provision, but the whole field of personal relations in courtship, in marriage and within the family - boy and girlfriend, husband and wife, parents and children, young and old'.(5)

Formal education is recognised as a vehicle to provide instruction on the means of ensuring stable family life. The core of Newsom's formula reappeared in *Ministry of Education's* handbook 'Health Education:1957', in which sex education is encouraged as a means to prevent 'broken homes'.

In 1964 the *Schools Council* was established to oversee and initiate curriculum innovation. The Cohen Report 'Health Education', of the same year, gave a general account of the knowledge base for health education in schools and society. It was highly critical both of school health education and of the Central Council for Health Education. They were said to be insufficiently informed by modern ideas about effective communication.

In the same year the *Church of England* Board of Education publication 'Sex Education in Schools' urged schools to 'accept some responsibility in sex education'.

The important 1967 *Plowden Report* 'Children and their Primary Schools', 'felt some reluctance about including a section on sex education'. Nevertheless a lengthy section was included. Significant excerpts include:

'We have no doubt that children's questions about sex ought to be answered plainly and truthfully whenever they are asked. Some questions will be repeated over the years and on each occasion the answer must satisfy. What is a proper and full answer for a six year old will not do for him four years later. The answers given must provide an acceptable and useable vocabulary for the child. This raises a difficulty. The 'popular' vocabulary, the four-letter words, is the one that the children will use clandestinely or openly among themselves. It is less taboo than it used to be , but most people would probably still consider it unacceptable for use in schools. Its associations are still too powerful. Circumlocution is often confusing, tends to be purely personal and have a sentimental, shame-faced sound. The scientific terms are really the only ones available.'(6)

Political Import

Up until the 1960s, those national reports dealing with sex/health education did not address particularly controversial issues. There was agreement on the self-evident merit of school instruction on matters of disease avoidance, reproduction, and preparation for sex roles suited to the single, dominant, desired family form. Legitimacy for the guidelines which filtered down to schools came largely from the unchallengeable authority of the medical profession, and to a lesser extent social scientists (eg. Bowlby's influence on Newsom Report) involved with government policy formation.

Within this formative period, centralised power is only beginning to be brought to bear on the subject. National regulations or guidelines are advisory and encouraging, though the subject is totally under the jurisdiction of the school. At this time the problem is perceived to be the need for greater exposure of the young to biological facts and 'a range of instructional activities aimed to encourage a healthier way of life'. The desired sexual morality and sex-role relationship is believed to be founded upon a scientific understanding of sexuality. Consequently, no problem presented itself in providing young people with the 'facts' of life other than the need to ration them to appropriate ages. Education might be described as a paternalistic process of enlightenment. Where 'power' operates in the politico-bureaucratic system, it takes the classical form of 'authority' where 'B complies with A because he recognises that A's command is reasonable in terms of his own values, either because its content is legitimate and reasonable, or because it is arrived at through a legitimate and reasonable procedure'.(7) The need for sex education was not contested even by the dominant religious authorities (other than Catholic). The problem was how such information could be conveyed in spite of the taboos which society had surrounded it with.

A number of developments would change this situation: the disintegration of the prevailing scientific conception of sexuality; politicisation of sexual roles and identities (feminism and sexual minorities); and the manifest failure of whatever passed for school sex education to halt the increase in teenage pregnancies and STDs. Henceforth, the 'preventive health' rationale for sex education (contraceptive education) would supersede what might be called the 'sexual socialisation' rationale.

This shift is evident in the pronouncements of the *British Medical Association*, representing the medical profession, where condemnation of teenage 'promiscuity' for the incidence of sexually transmitted diseases gave way to hard-headed advocacy of contraceptive education, and the defence of the right of young adolescents to contraceptive counselling from their doctors.

Changes in the social mores of adolescents during the 1960s were to affect the 'political' component of health/sex education administration. The free availability of contraception and the arrival of the Pill dissociated sex not only from reproduction but marriage itself. In this period, sexuality was given new significance as a more explicit dimension of life and a vehicle of political change. The 1967 *Sexual Offences Act* had incorporated Wolfenden's decriminalisation of male homosexual acts conducted in private by two consenting adults, expanding, along with the 1967 *Abortion Act*, the scope of sex education into the most controversial areas. The adolescent population became an increasing focus of political attention in respect of pregnancy rates, STDs, and subsequently, abortions. Controllers of the Media have wielded a negative power throughout the recent history of sex education in refusing to expose the television-watching public of any age to contraceptives, though the threat of AIDS has altered this attitude by the late-1980s.

The *Roman Catholic Church* stands isolated and defiant in its refusal to countenance anything other than a traditionalistic, anti-('artificial') contraceptive sex education within schools under its control; its influence on British society is also manifested in organisations (eg. anti-abortion movements such as 'Life' and the Society for the Protection of the Unborn Child (SPUC), and by outspoken Roman Catholics inside and outside of Parliament (eg. Victoria Gillick).

1968-78

This period sees the rising influence of interest-groups competing with the medical establishment's input to school health/sex education. Independent 'traditionalist' and 'progressive' movements emerge in competition for influence over how sexuality enters the classroom.

The subject is recognised by the authorities to be more complex than had been previously thought, demanding expertise which medical authorities alone could not or did not offer. This was dealt with nationally in two ways: firstly, in response to the perceived need for preventive health education, in 1968, the *Health Education Council* replaced The Central Council for Health Education, after 40 years existence, with a much enlarged 'education and training' section. Correspondingly, the *Department of Education and Science's* more comprehensive 'Handbook of Health Education' (1968) replaced the old Ministry of Education handbook, including in it a chapter on 'School and the Future Parent' which suggested that the study of literature is as important as the biological sciences in helping to form 'standards of value and attitude to sex'.

Secondly, in the face of an evolving and complex field, no criteria existed for the training of teachers. The government of the day was sympathetic to bona fide independent organisations stepping in where 'official' means were lacking.

The first major expression of the political controversies to come appeared in the form of the 1976 *House of Lords* debate on sex education and the public funding of the Family Planning Association as a bona fide 'expert' resource in this field sub-contracted by government (see Chapter 3). Although the government of the day defended its financial (and ideological) support for the FPA, a vociferous Parliamentary movement in opposition to the current political management of state sex education presented itself.

1976 *Schools Council Working Paper 57*: 'Health Education in Secondary Schools'. This working paper from the Schools Council identified a number of sex education topics in its definition of health education, and reviewed several different patterns of curriculum organisation and teaching methods appropriate to providing it.

1976 *Department of Health and Social Security* : Court Report 'Fit for the Future'. This report on the organisation of the child health services endorsed the view that health education in schools should be seen as an important facet of preventive medicine.

1977 *Department of Health and Social Security Report*: 'Prevention and Health: Everybody's Business'. This broadly based report sought to give a higher status and priority to health promotion and disease prevention, and a section on health education includes these comments:

'The Health and Education departments accept the value of providing sex education in schools. This is, however, a sensitive subject in which any school contemplating the use of controversial teaching material or speakers should tell parents what it intends to do....(sex education) forms part of wider programmes of education in lasting personal relationships, and (it) should seek to relate factual knowledge to the individual sense of personal responsibility: it should not be confined to physiological aspects and contraception. The emphasis on the importance of responsible and loving relationships is therefore to be welcomed'.

1977 *Schools Council HEC Publication*: 'Health Education 5-13'. This was a comprehensive set of teaching materials and guidelines, produced initially by the Schools Council, and later in partnership with the Health Education Council. An extensive section on education and personal relationships was included. The Schools Council's annotated selection of publications and teaching aids 'Relationships and Sexuality' (1982) prepared for the 'Health Education Project 13-18' recommends approximately 80 publications and audio-visual aids.

1977 *Department of Education and Science Report*: 'Health Education in Schools'. This replaced the 1968 Handbook of Health Education, and includes a full chapter on sex education. On this occasion the DES recognised that there are no 'standard answers' to the Who?, When?, What?, and Where? of sex education(pg 109-119).

1978 *Her Majesty's Inspectorate Report Curriculum* 11-16: 'Health Education in the Secondary School'. This was one of a set of reports which Her Majesty's Inspectorate for Schools issued as contributions to what became known as 'The Great Debate' on education in Britain, which was just beginning at that time. It argued strongly for a place for health education, as an aspect of education for attitudes, as well as for facts.

The *National Marriage Guidance Council* was with the FPA one of the two major 'bona fide' organisations which offered their services to the school system. Since the 1950s, the NMGC had been concerned with teaching about marital roles as a basis for family stability. Wallis notes that its early popular booklet 'How to treat a Young Wife' (1951) was concerned with the sexual preconditions of marital well-being, laying stress on the man's development of his wife's sexual potentialities: an emergent theme of sex education material aimed at older girls and young women. Nevertheless, the NMGC was essentially a marital counselling organisation which had a restricted role in providing sex education in the classroom. As the subject became oriented more around the management of sexuality in adolescence (pregnancy prevention and the avoidance of STDs), so the NMGC handed over to the expertise of the FPA. Ultimately the NMGC would cease to undertake school visits for the purposes of sex education. Due to a reconsideration of its policy on pre-marital education, the Family Planning Association has had a central role during this period and is dealt with separately as a postscript to this chapter.

The similar-minded *National Viewers' and Listeners' Association* regards contemporary school sex education as a violation of the ideal relationship between parent and child, and opposes any form of sex education which does not place biological information within a traditional moral dimension.

Political Import (see figure 3 page 80)

The governmental management of school sex education has necessarily involved the two ministries of health and education whose ideological differences and orientations have strongly influenced the development of this subject; something which is likely to be the case in all countries. In the case of the FPA role, the initial contacts and cooperation with government were almost exclusively via the Department of Health and Social Security, whose responsibility was not only family planning but the 'education' of health personnel. Due to its more scientifically grounded 'preventive medicine' rationale, the DHSS has been willing and able to be more 'progressive' and liberal in its approach to public education regarding (sexual) moral issues than its more conservative and ideologically sensitive sister Department of Education and Science.

The control of the DES over the educational system has created organisational limits to the delivery of health education into the classroom, and inevitably produces a degree of bureaucratic demarcation and even rivalry when it comes to publicly controversial issues. The DHSS-funded FPA educational work could not extend to school teachers because of the potential conflict with DES jurisdiction over funds for training for this profession. The DES has never supported the sex education work of the FPA as the DHSS has, although Her Majesty's inspectors have lent support in various ways.

It may be concluded from the above that the moral-ideological persuasions of senior civil servants directing these Ministries, rather than their political masters, will decide the degree to which the ministerial machine will be used to facilitate or block the development of the subject.

In this period, the development of sex education through the work of the quasi-autotomous non-governmental organisations, such as the Schools Council, HEC and the work of the independent FPA was a result of the liberal persuasions of otherwise inaccessible and invisible DHSS senior civil

FIG 3.

**POLITICAL AND ADMINISTRATIVE MANAGEMENT OF SCHOOL SEX
EDUCATION IN ENGLAND 1968-1977**

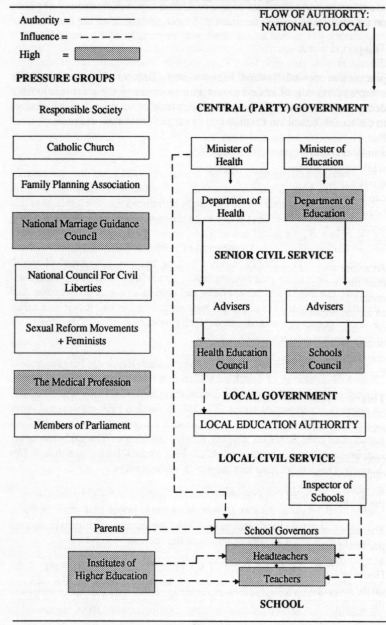

servants. Any differences of ideological persuasion or distrust between the senior policy makers of the two bureaucracies will create a great impediment to any independent organisation which must rely upon the cooperation of both on the same issue for a programme of education to be taken forward.

This period is characterised by increasing demand for expertise which simply did not exist in this new field. Consequently, control over the educational process was open and flexible. The government departments resorted to those sources of training which had some legitimacy in the society in order to fill a demand which it could not itself fill. Sub-contracting the task of sex education to the Health Education Council (HEC), which in turn sub-contracted to the Family Planning Information Service of the FPA, has permitted successive administrations to fund the independent contraceptive sex education approach while insulating themselves organisationally by means of the buffer of the quasi-autonomous HEC. While acting as no more than a conduit for funds, it can nevertheless absorb opposition to the FPA which otherwise might have been directed at the government Ministry of Health. The organisational separation between the FPA's information service and its (sex) education unit increased this insulation.(8)

At a time when progressivism in sex education meant nothing more complex than the need to get more 'facts' over to pupils in order that they have the means to make decisions and adjust 'unhealthy' behaviour, the priority was to secure personnel who were able to overcome the taboos of open discussion of these sexual facts of life with people of different ages. It was this uncontroversial 'technical' requirement in training which the FPA was commissioned by government to deliver to the educational system, along with family planning (quasi-medical) expertise.

This arrangement successfully served the purposes both of those commissioning, and those supplying this sex education training to health and educational staff. Though the broader legitimacy of such training was taken for granted by both sides which opposition remained muted or small scale (see Chapter 3). In more recent times, under the impact of more vocal opposition, the full moral-political significance of what can and must be included in the term 'sex education' has been realised by parliamentarians and the public.

The scope of action of the Health Education Council shifted with the wider political climate over sex education. In times of controversy, it is singled out as a primary government point of reference on policy and practice (see 1976 House of Lords debate). Yet it has never sought to develop an explicit policy on the subject which might form the basis of a national curriculum. Moreover, the guidelines it has produced are based upon the broad 'consensus' of the teaching profession rather than on any expert authority. It is not preoccupied with this subject as a priority compared with other health education issues, nor has any government recommended that it become an authority on this subject. The HEC has embarked upon guidelines for sex education, such as through its resource list of sex education materials endorsed for school use (the Schools Health Education Project). However, political interference in the content of acceptable sex education materials endorsed by the HEC led it simply to cease updating this list as a service to schools.

Whether by accident or design, the political structure governing sex education turned out to be a series of sub-contracting operations *which has served to remove responsibility from any single body*. The School Curriculum Development Committee - which replaced the Schools Council - is deprived of policy-making powers within curriculum innovation, and is now no more concerned with sex education per se than the HEC. Similarly, *Her Majesty's School Inspectors* report on schools, and though not simply functionaries for the DES (whose heads are advisers to the Minister), do not constitute any independent power in curriculum development either.

1977-1986 (See figure 4 page 86)

This period, saw the beginnings of the dismantling of the sub-contracting arrangements with quasi-and non-govenmental organisations. Its highlight came with the 1986 *Education Act* in which the government chose to instruct local authorities how the subject was to be presented henceforth. It can be seen as the first stage in removal of decision-making powers from a local government entirely.

The 1979 *Department of Education and Science Report*: 'Aspects of Secondary Education in England' blamed: 'lack of leadership and agreed policies' for deficiencies in the quality and quantity of sex education in schools.

In the 1980 *Education Act* (Section 8), consideration was given during the passage of this Act to whether parents should have the right to withdraw their children from sex education classes (as with religious education). But it was decided that this should not be permitted as sex education is not a compulsory subject.

1981 *Education (School Information) Regulation* required Local Education Authorities and School Governors to publish information about 'the manner and context in which education as respects sexual matters is given'.(9)

1981 *Department of Education and Science* 'The School Curriculum' stated:

'There are also some essential constituents of the school curriculum which are often identified as subjects but which are as likely to feature in a variety of courses and programmes and may be more effectively covered if they are distributed across the curriculum. These concern personal and social development, and can conveniently be grouped under the headings of moral education, health education (including sex education) and preparation for parenthood and family life' (1981 para 23)....'preparation for parenthood and family life should help pupils to recognise the importance of those human relationships which sustain and are sustained by family life and the demands and duties that fall on parents.' (para 25)

1986 (July) *Her Majesty's Inspectorate*: 'Health Education 5-16' This discussion document appeared as one of a series on 'Curriculum Matters'. More than 6 of its 30 pages are devoted to sex education. However, issues of controversy such as homosexuality are left strictly to local authorities, schools and their governors to adjudicate on, with the proviso that all shades of opinion be taken into account. In this respect they cannot in any real sense be described as 'guidelines' to practitioners.

1986 (August) *Department of Education and Science:* Draft Circular 'Sex Education at School'. This document was widely published by the DES, and sent out for discussion to a range of national bodies. While incorporating some HMI suggestions, it differs on several points.

The House of Commons debate on the sex education clause of the 1986 *Education Bill* sees a 'knee-jerk' defence of the status quo by the political opposition (see chapter 3).

1986 (December) *Education Act* (Chp 61). This Act changed the constitution and powers of governing bodies of schools, and makes several specifications for sex education as follows:

Para 18

(2) The articles of government for every such school shall provide for it to be the duty of the governing body,

a) to consider separately (while having regard to the local education authority's statement under Section 17 of this Act) the question whether sex education should form part of the secular curriculum for the school; and

b) to make and keep up to date, a separate written statement -

(i) of their policy with regard to the content and organisation of the relevant part of the curriculum; or

(ii) where they conclude that sex education should not form part of the secular curriculum, of that conclusion.

Part III (3) The articles of government for every such school shall provide for it to be the duty of the governing body -

a) when considering the matters mentioned in subsections (1) and (2) above, to do so in consultation with the head teacher and to have regard -

(i) to any representations which are made to them, with regard to any of those matters, by any persons connected with the community served by the school; and

(ii) to any such representations which are made to them by the chief officer of police and which are connected with his responsibilities

(b) to consult the authority before making or varying any statement under subsection (1) above; and

c) to furnish the authority and head teacher with an up to date copy of any statement under this section.

Paragraph 46: Sex Education

The local education authority by whom any county, voluntary or special school is maintained, and the governing body and head teacher of the school, shall take such steps as are reasonably practicable to secure that where sex education is given to any registered pupils at the school it is given in such a manner as to encourage those pupils to have due regard to moral considerations and the value of family life (effective from Jan. 7/87).

Paragraph 31:

1) Subject to subsections (7) and (8) below, the articles of government for every county, voluntary and maintained special school shall provide for it to be the duty of the governing body to hold a meeting once in every school year ('the annual parents meeting') which is open to:

a) all parents of registered pupils at the school;

b) the head teacher; and

c) such other persons as the governing body may invite.

2) The purpose of the meeting shall be to provide an opportunity for discussion of :

a) the governors' report; and

b) the discharge of the governing body, the head teacher and the local education authority of their functions in relation to the school (effective from Jan. 7/87).

In 1979, the *Brook Advisory Centres (which was was set up as a separate organisation to the FPA in 1964 in order to undertake the more contentious role of providing family planning to young unmarried* women) produced a pamphlet entitled: 'A Look at Safe Sex'. This was subsequently questioned in the House of Commons and now bears an instruction from the Department of Education and Science outlawing its use in schools on the grounds of its directness in giving information to the young. DHSS financial support for the BAC is increasingly questioned in Parliament on the grounds of its sex education materials. Politicians continue to adopt the role of monitors of the country's morals using Parliament itself as the arena in which sex education texts are scrutinised.

Such is the power of moral discredit that one vocal member of parliament can threaten the entire grant to an organisation and none is willing to risk political standing to defend a sex education organisation. Moreover, the DHSS and DES resort to an 'index' of prohibited sex education texts is more likely a response to the demands of their political masters fear of this moral minority, than to create a curriculum 'within the broad directive of right and wrong which society gives' as the Crowther report put it.

Political Import

Towards the end of the 1970s, the system of governmental sub-contracting in sex education curriculum design was reversed. Traditionalist members of government, aided by the media, demanded that the government act to curb threatened moral discredit to high government, itself. However, it should not be presumed that legislation which appeared in the mid-1980s was an expression of desire for a new form of sex education. Rather, such measures might be understood as means by which government could allay or divert criticism to other bodies in the political management structure.

Thus, through the 1981 *Education (Schools Information) Act,* local education authorities and school governors were not compelled or directed to alter the sex education they were offering schools, but merely to expose it to public scrutiny, thereby forcing a self-censorship on what the latter might feel would be subjected to public criticism. This astute political measure does not place government in the role of being 'anti-progressive', merely 'democratic', as

FIG 4.

**POLITICAL AND ADMINISTRATIVE MANAGEMENT OF SCHOOL SEX
EDUCATION IN ENGLAND 1977-1986**

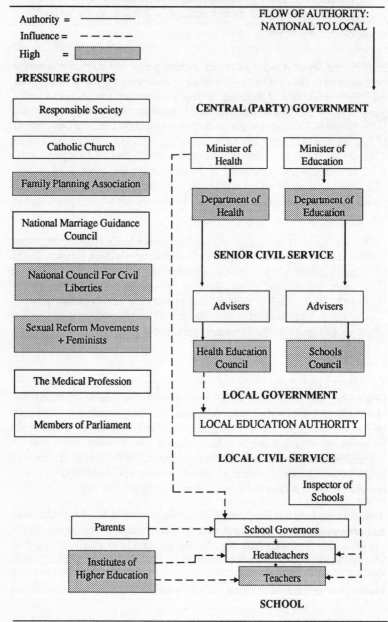

the pretence may now be upheld not only that parents have been brought into the scrutinising process, but are made (partially) responsible for it.

A *National Council of Women of Great Britain* report: 'Sex Education: Whose Responsibility?' revealed that by 1984 there was still a lack of communication between parents and schools with a 'significant number' of schools only providing the legal minimum in the way of informing and consulting parents. Such is the climate created by a power structure organised for the purposes more of censorship than progress.

With the inclusion of head teachers in the 1986 Act proposals, a counterbalance is formed with the schools governing body, thus making each liable to the other in terms of avoiding moral discredit through use of 'unacceptable materials'. The government has at a stroke made impotent the only sources of professional sex education curriculum design, replacing these with self-regulating amateur bodies devoid of any guidance.

The sex education clause of the 1986 Education Act making local education authorities responsible for schools conforming to 'family values' in their sex education classes, appears at first glance to be a triumph for the right in pushing back 'progressivism'. However, the careful wording of the regulation reveals itself to be an astute political mechanism which permits the conservative government to 'appear' to be responding to its own right- wing, while leaving the definition of the family implicit opening the doors to any number of interpretations of what might constitute a 'family'. It turns out to be a largely empty amendment, if not placating, keeping at bay right and left by responding to their concerns simultaneously.

This clause turns out to be merely a device used by the government for the purposes of political self-protection from the charge from its own right wing of indifference to the issue (moral discredit). It serves not only to confuse rather than help resolve problems of sex education ideology, but encourages fruitless future charges of school non-compliance according to the interpretation placed on the term 'family' and even takeover of power by one interest group or another. The threat which 'moral discredit' poses leads one to suspect that no government is ever likely to directly repeal the law, in spite of the confusion it has created, on the grounds that they would not wish to appear to be in any way 'anti-family'. They may, however, create new legislation which simply supercedes it.

On this occasion the school governing board and head teacher are placed in the firing line. It remains to be seen whether the representative Associations of governors and head teachers will be willing to defend their members in this field.

In addition to teachers, medical and other academic professionals, have been excluded from the decision-making educational 'establishment', presuming their voice in curriculum development organisations such as the Schools Council was ever heard. The right of teachers to provide the sex education of *their* choice is now regulated by the albeit inexperienced school governing bodies, which must of necessity supervise on the side of caution - the spectre of exposure to moral discredit rules the day.

In earlier periods the entire political process by which teachers would give sex education of a certain form was based on 'sapiential authority' (authority by virtue of knowledge) - that teachers would willingly respond to regulations and directions from higher in the political system *because* they are felt to be legitimate and reasonable in terms of teachers' own values. This cannot be said to pertain in this re-assertion of power. It must be concluded that the government is less concerned with the quality of teaching than with what they must not give because of the threat this poses to the moral credibility of the political management *in the eyes of those who pose a threat to the government's position*. What is lost is willing teacher participation and creativity - the only real basis for sex education in the absence of any examinable orthodoxy.

Educational authorities and their advisory bodies in the 1970s *hoped* that teachers would be assisted in what they were provided with to provide the best possible education. Now, there is no longer concern about the quality of sex education given, only its propriety. The 1987 regulations are less designed to enhance the equality of sex education than to ensure political survival of the control mechanism. Teachers can in this regime simply choose to do nothing, and only head teachers have the power to monitor this.

Sexual minority groups have been morally discredited by a combination of real and imaginary scandals fuelled by the media. Teachers openly supporting minority sexual rights have been discredited in the same process (through individual exposes, gay teacher groups etc.). Teachers as a profession pose no threat whatsoever to the government on this issue.

The FPA relied partly on its history as *the* national family planning authority, and through this identity established its influence with its education clientele: teachers and health professionals. But this power base has now been weakened. In terms of influence over sex education, the FPA has also been marginalised, mainly because it no longer controls a 'scarce resource' which the government *needs*. This is not so much because there are now alternative sources of sex education training but, one suspects, because the government of the 1980s is less sure about either the value of such education as 'enlightenment' for its own sake, in a 'sexually pluralist' society, or the positive contribution such education as exists makes to teenage pregnancy rates.

1987

April 1987 The *Health Education Council* is dissolved, responsibilities for health education brought within the higher levels of the Department of Health and Social Security.

1987 (July) *Department of Education and Science* : 'The National Curriculum 5-16'. This consultation document proposes a comprehensive reform of school curriculum, with (for example, in years 4 and 5 of secondary school) 90% of the time devoted to foundation subjects - English, Maths, Science, Technology, Modern Languages, History, Geography, Arts, Physical education; with 'additional subjects' fitted in to the remaining 10%. Sex education is not mentioned, but 'health education' is commented on as follows:

18. In addition, there are a number of subjects or themes such as health education and use of information technology, which can be taught through other subjects. For example, biology can contribute to learning about health education, and the health theme will give an added dimension to teaching about biology. It is proposed that such subjects or themes should be taught through the foundation subjects, so that they can be accommodated within the curriculum but without crowding out the essential subjects.

1987 (September) *Department of Education and Science* Circular: 'Sex Education at School'. This differs very markedly from the draft circular issued a year before. It incorporates the requirements of the 1986 Education Act, and emphasises the moral and legal frameworks for sex education. Topics on which it presents new and definitive proscriptions are homosexuality, and contraceptive advice to pupils under 16 years old. Noteworthy excerpts are as follows:

A Moral Framework for Sex Education:

18. Section 46 of the Education (No 2) Act 1986 requires that, 'The local education authority by whom any county, voluntary or special school is maintained, and the governing body and head teacher of the school, shall take such steps as are reasonably practicable to secure that where sex education is given to any registered pupils at the school it is given in such a manner as to encourage those pupils to have due regard to moral considerations and the value of family life'.

19. The Secretary of State considers that the aims of a programme of sex education should be to present facts in an objective and balanced manner so as to enable pupils to comprehend the range of sexual attitudes and behaviour in present day society; to know what is and what is not legal; to consider their own attitudes, and to make informed, reasoned and responsible decisions about the attitudes they will adopt both while they are at school and in adulthood. Teaching about the physical aspects of sexual behaviour should be set within a clear moral framework in which pupils are encouraged to consider the importance of self-restraint, dignity and respect for themselves and others, and helped to recognise the physical, emotional and moral risks of casual and promiscuous sexual behaviour. Schools should foster a recognition that both sexes should have responsibility in sexual matters. Pupils should be helped to appreciate the benefits of stable married and family life and the responsibilities of parenthood.

20. Schools have a responsibility to ensure that pupils understand those aspects of the law which relate to sexual activity. Pupils should understand three things in particular, which are that:

i. except in certain very restricted circumstances, it is a criminal offence for a man or boy to have sexual intercourse with a girl under 16, irrespective of whether she consents;

ii. homosexual acts (defined as buggery or gross indecency) between males constitute a criminal offence unless both parties have attained the age of 21 and the acts are committed with the consent of both in private (ie. where only two parties are present); and

iii. it is an offence to make an indecent assault on a person; and a girl or boy under 16 cannot in law give any consent which would prevent an act being an assault for the purpose of this offence.

21. Schools cannot, in general, avoid tackling controversial sexual matters, such as contraception and abortion, by reason of their sensitivity. Pupils may well ask questions about them and schools should be prepared to offer balanced and factual information and to acknowledge the major ethical issues involved. Where schools are founded on specific religious principles this will have a direct bearing on the manner in which such subjects are presented.

22. There is no place in any school in any circumstances for teaching which advocates homosexual behaviour, which presents it as the 'norm', or which encourages homosexual experimentation by pupils. Indeed, encouraging or procuring homosexual acts by pupils who are under the age of consent is a criminal offence. It must also

be recognised that for many people, including members of various religious faiths, homosexual practice is not morally acceptable, and deep offence may be caused to them if the subject is not handled with sensitivity by teachers if discussed in the classroom.

Advice For Pupils Under 16:

25. It is important to distinguish between, on the one hand, the school's function of providing education generally about sexual matters on the basis described above and, on the other, counselling and advice to individual pupils, particularly if this relates to their own sexual behaviour. Good teachers have always taken a pastoral interest in the welfare and well-being of pupils. But this function should never trespass on the proper exercise of parental rights and responsibilities.

26. On the specific question of the provision of contraceptive advice to girls under 16, the general rule must be that giving an individual pupil advice on such matters without parental knowledge or consent would be an inappropriate exercise of a teacher's professional responsibilities, and could, depending on the circumstances, amount to a criminal offence. The provision of contraceptive advice and treatment was addressed by the House of Lords' judgement in the Gillick case. The House of Lords found that, while it should be most unusual for a doctor to provide such a service to a child under 16 without parental knowledge or consent, there were circumstances, described in the judgements, where he or she would be justified in doing so. These circumstances hinged essentially upon the nature and context of medical advice and treatment in connection with the supply and use of contraceptive devices. They have no parallel in school education.

27. A teacher approached by a pupil for advice on these or other aspects of sexual behaviour should, wherever possible, encourage the pupil to seek advice from his or her parents. Where the circumstances are such as to lead the teacher to believe that the pupil has embarked upon , or is contemplating, a course of conduct which is likely to place him or her in moral or physical danger, or in breach of the law, the teacher has a general duty to warn the pupil of the risks involved. Whether the teacher should take the matter further, by informing the head teacher, and whether the head teacher should consider involving the pupil's parents, the specialist support services, or the local education authority, will depend on the particular circumstances involved and the professional judgement of the staff.

Political Import (see figure 5 page 93)

During the 1980s, the relatively independent status of the DHSS-funded Health Education Council has been eroded to the point that, by 1987 it was fundamentally re-structured as the Health Education Authority - a component of the NHS management system. The government's decision to absorb this body within a more centralised managerial system was in part due to disagreement between the HEC's and the government's line of thinking on certain health issues. However, it is unlikely that disagreement over appropriate sex education figured very greatly in this (for example, the government grant to the Family Planning Association has remained intact). Nevertheless, sex did play some role in the rhetoric of transformation, as the government justification for the dissolution of the original Council was based on the perceived need to create 'a more effective agency for AIDS prevention'.

In a similar process, the professional advisory body, the Schools Council, has also lost independence in terms of funding and content through its re-establishment as the School Curriculum Development Council (SCDC); a body which has no role in the decision-making process but is restricted to the collection of curriculum development information, the suitability of which is decided elsewhere. (The SCDC is now also abolished.)

The *National Curriculum* proposals, in the form of a Bill, have marginalised health as well as sex education to the point that it is no longer included by name in consultation documents. Where sex education is mentioned, as in the DES circular, it presents curriculum guidelines in which the substance is secondary to what is to be proscribed. It is interesting to note that what it does say implies that the school population is already likely to have acquired the kind of knowledge which earlier sex education models might have proposed to teach; and that it must merely be informed of what society (the law) will and will not tolerate before punitive measures are applied. It expects that knowledge be given in a 'neutral' fashion, though it offers warnings to those teachers who might wish to stray into discussing minority sexual politics. This represents an example of the political mobilisation of bias - one manifestation of power, where barriers are constructed to the continued public airing of policy conflicts. This circular acts to foreclose discussion on the content of sex education by threat of moral discredit through the rule of law as an unnegotiable given.

Moreover, in spite of the lip-service paid to the importance of the subject for personal development, it is returned to a place in the curriculum in which it began its career: biology. Using the pretext of the need to protect the integrity of the 'essential foundation subjects' in the curriculum, the Government appears to be an attempting to close Pandora's Box, by limiting access to the

FIG 5.

POLITICAL AND ADMINISTRATIVE MANAGEMENT OF SCHOOL SEX EDUCATION IN ENGLAND 1987

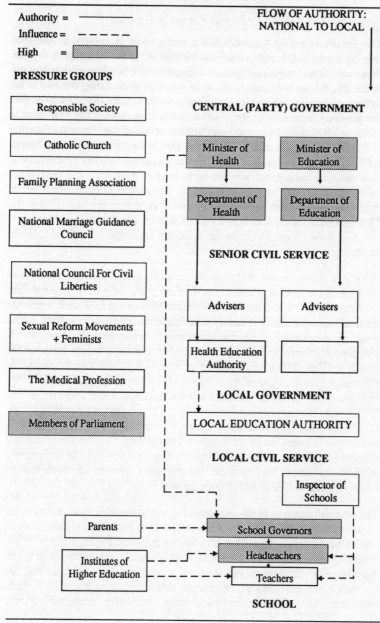

full scientific and political approach to the subject by enclosing it within one part of the curriculum believed to be uncontentious.

Postscript: The Role of the Family Planning Association

The Family Planning Association has had a more controversial career in gaining the bona fide status awarded the NMGC in the educational system. Its national status originated through its control of the family planning services of the UK, whose political significance was hightened during the 1960s due to the population issue. In fact, its political respectability had been secured in the previous decade, with the visit of Minister of Health, Ian MacLeod in 1955. In 1966, the Minister of Health had announced that 'general education in family planning is a most important part of health education' (Circular 5/66). In the 1960s, Sir Keith Joseph commissioned a survey by the FPA to find out why people did not use birth control methods - the first direct government interest in the Association. Through the involvement of its volunteer workers with pre-marital as well as contraceptive counselling , the FPA moved naturally towards sex education proper. However, its national status as (one) 'expert' organisation in sex education was secured more indirectly.

In 1972, The Department of Health and Social Security was collaborating with the FPA in the process of absorbing the family planning clinic network into the National Health Service. Henceforth, the FPA would be funded to provide information and training in family planning to those entering the NHS. Good political cooperation with the government department resulted in this independent charity being funded to provide courses in family planning for health visitors (5,000 being trained at a cost of £250,000). A subsequent evaluation questionnaire of these health visitors revealed that 54% did not feel they could easily discuss matters of sex and birth control with clients. The DHSS was informed of the problem along with plans by FPA staff to begin (in 1977) an 'experimental' teaching programme in this uncharted field. With few human resources and little theoretical foundation, the FPA aimed to begin the process of heath visitor sex education. Once established, the Department of Health continued funding these 'sex education' courses for health visitors to the extent of £70,000-£75,000 per annum.

The essential function of this new teaching was to discover by experiment the means to teach communication skills sufficient to deal with a highly personal and embarrassing subject. This priority has remained the cornerstone of the 'experiential' focus of FPA Education Unit courses for the teaching and health professionals. In view of the specially sensitive subject of teaching, the courses were designed to be purely voluntary, though the FPA soon discovered that many reluctant health visitors were being compelled to attend.

This is significant both because of the importance which this training was felt to have by health authorities, and because it reveals what a scarce resource, the 'expertise' the FPA was believed to have, was.

Subsequently, the FPA was requested to help fill the felt need for sex education in schools, by working with NMGC personnel in covering the contraceptive field. By this time there was some anxiety within the FPA that FPA volunteers were entering this potentially controversial area without any standardised programme of training or control by the Association. At the expense of some conflict within the Association, a training programme was eventually developed.

1970 marked the beginning of the FPA work in schools, themselves, with staff needing not only to train those representing the Association in this role, but designing the very training courses themselves from scratch. As a result, the approach to sexuality per se was founded upon an intuitive, 'progressive' ideology (suited to the times) rather than any systematic sexological foundation or political approach to the subject. The theoretical vacuum was filled by adaptation of the kind of psychodynamic person-centred approaches which had such an influence on (particularly USA) family social work during the late 1950s and early 1960s.

The early programmes were conducted throughout Britain (5-6 per annum) with the permission of the local education authorities. In turn, social services departments requested 'training' for social work students in order that they could deal with any sexual component of problems. Again, the Department of Health provided the funds to establish courses for social workers, which they examined and found acceptable.

The Rationale of the FPA Education Unit

The struggle to take the FPA from its 'safe' base in family planning into sex education was achieved at a cost of some internal disagreement. In view of the controversial nature of this new venture, the education unit remains separate in its operation from the central advisory and information service of the FPA. This separation therefore has a strategic purpose in respect of the FPA proper, its medical volunteer and Ministerial support, *vis-à-vis* the education unit.

Those directing this expansion of FPA activities from birth control (with its unambiguous 'preventive medicine'- health rationale) to adolescent sex education (with its far more complex and controversial rationales : for example, psycho-sexual well-being) perceived correctly that education based purely upon factual contraceptive information would not and could not be tolerated in view of the moral consequences of such activity. The realm of education in (sexual) *relationships* was no less of a minefield than contraceptive information. Like sex reformers in Europe, FPA pioneers were united in their desire to eliminate guilt and fear from sexual matters. Work in family planning clinics revealed this psychological burden which often manifested itself in sexual dysfunction, and which the medical profession was not concerned with or or unable to help.

The philosophy adopted rests upon implicit assumptions about the nature of human sexuality rather than an explicit elaboration of scientific theories - that sexuality is at root a positive force, and that all sexualities can be catered for in a context of mutual love and respect, and that moral values are rational and self-evident. According to degree of maturity, everyone has a right to 'full, objective' information about sexuality, and that for sex educators to be qualified they should have a 'full knowledge of the basic facts of human sexuality', although this is not the main purpose of the teaching provided. The code of sexual ethics delivered through the teaching courses has included the following principles: acceptance of masturbation as harmless, (responsible) pre-marital sexual activity through avoidance of pregnancy by using contraceptives, and (implicit) support for homosexual rights.

The demand for 'qualifications' in this uncharted field from health and educational authorities overshadowed the fact that the UKFPA (along with other European FPAs) drew from what scientific evidence was available a liberal value position regarding sexuality, human rights and responsibilities. The legitimacy of the FPA as the national training resource for this subject lay rather upon a reputation grounded in the family planning clinic, service-delivery field rather than in the theory and practice of sex education. Consequently, the FPA training courses have been eclectic in their choice of materials (in 1982 the FPA's booklist would detail 31 commercial publications on sex education) and have continued to focus more upon the teaching of communication skills rather than the 'knowledge' referred to above, concentrating less upon the substance of the subject and the moral issues raised.

If, as proposed here, this has been a weakness in the defences of the FPA programme, it did not reveal itself in a period sympathetic to progressive discovery and experimentation. The Department of Health itself approved of the FPA sex education policy, a significant fact in the quite different political climate of the 1980s, when more anti-progressive sentiments hold sway. Curiously, the FPA faced its first public scandal over government-funded courses for the handicapped, as it appears that some critics were unable to come to terms with the idea of handicapped people having sexual needs or problems. In more recent times, following the FPA pathfinding, some institutions for the training of teachers provide their own training courses (circa 10% non-obligatory), as well as some LEAs and Curriculum Development Centres. Even though school teachers have rarely made up more than 15% of the attenders of FPA courses in its history, it is fair to say that this independent organisation has had a significant influence upon the style of sex education delivered in the classroom. The FPA has been such a prime mover in this field that many of its 'graduates' have gone on to teach others in coordination with Local Education Authorities.

The movement of 'progressive' organisations such as the FPA into the field of sex education increased the resistance of counter-movements such as The Responsible Society (whose ideas were given a parliamentary voice in the 1976 House of Lords debate on sex education. Part of the spectrum of 'anti-permissive', Christian- based organisations concerned with public morality, the Responsible Society was inaugurated in 1971 as a 'watchdog' to monitor the content of sex education, and to 'advance the education of the public in the United Kingdom in matters of personal responsibility with particular reference to sexual relationships'.(10) It exists to combat 'the steady increases over recent years in venereal diseases, unwanted pregnancies, abortions, illegitimate births and other consequences of promiscuous behaviour, especially among teenagers' (11) which it sees as 'long term threats to stable and loving relationships' ... 'most of the teaching aids currently available for use in the classroom are amoral in approach and others are frankly subversive'.(12) In the 1980s, the FPA continues its work in sex education training with the support on which it has traditionally relied, though in defiance of a range of opposition forces which court their own government allies.

Conclusion

The post war history of sex education may be described with reference to the rationales which have dominated its phases, and the political management structures which dialectically relate to them. The first prescribed a reinforcement programme of socialisation into the sex roles and obligations which were believed to be normal, natural and healthy for the individual and society alike. The major problem to be confronted was the psychological taboo to teaching and conscious learning.

This rationale was eclipsed through changing social conditions, mores and contraceptive technology. The preventive-health rationale was a less ambitious organisation of education to create sexual responsibility through contraceptive awareness. If sexual socialisation could not be influenced by education, it was nevertheless necessary to provide the young with the information necessary to protect their health. Even in this second phase, the FPA in particular managed to retain a reasonable monopoly on the knowledge required. This rationale was subjected to criticism from the right, firstly, because of its 'technical' over moral priority, and secondly, because of its 'pupil-centred' approach to value-acquisition, in which young people arrive at their own considered decisions on issues with the assistance of a 'neutral' teacher.

In the last phase, the rapid development of our scientific understanding of sexuality led inexorably to a rationale which might be termed: 'education for responsible sexual self-determination'. This rationale has gained notoriety through the willingness of some teachers and local authorities to broaden the subject to include non-procreative relationships, sexual discrimination etc. Although its impact on classroom teaching is unknown, it is this which the present administration has taken steps to forbid in an attempt to re-establish a more ideologicially palatable physical-health rationale. The collapse of the 'factual' basis for scientific sexology, which has transformed this subject during the 1970s (with the addition of a critical-political dimension) suggests that the political rationale for sex education will not so easily be suppressed. (See Chapter 3 'Fact and Value').

The development of this difficult field in a spirit of consensus has been shown to have had an insecure foundation in the 1970s. At this time, progressive elements were encouraged by government, while moral considerations, and ultimately opposition alliances were disregarded. In spite of the sub-contracting process, the dominance of the progressive autonomous, semi-autonomous and government bodies, which became established during the late 1960s and early 1970s, depended more upon the support of the higher governmental authorities (central DHSS), rather than the lower educational ones (school governors; head teachers). It has been suggested that the alliance between governmental authorities and interest groups which prevailed in the 1960s and 1970s sowed the seeds of the their own destruction in this respect.

With the mandate given to the Right at the turn of the decade, this narrow legitimacy was removed. In a climate in which anti-'progressive' forces now have the floor, the Conservative government is wary of internal as well as external criticism. For the sake of self-protection against the threat of moral discredit, the government has terminated or re-negotiated many of the earlier sub-contractual arrangements, shifting power over the future of school sex education away from traditionally 'progressive' bodies.

Thus, it might be argued that the government has clarified and reconstituted the lines of power governing the political management of sex education to suit its own political rather than purely educational purposes. In the process, the means by which power is exercised in the management and development of the subject has shifted from genuine 'authority' to a system of constraint, coercion, centralisation and (self-) policing. It is difficult to see how the new arrangement - the power base set up between head teachers and governors - can function effectively if this creates a barrier between the head teacher and the classroom teacher. Should the broader moral-political climate swing back towards the left in the future, it may be seen that this government has also established its sex education mandate on an equally inadequate foundation, by alienating rather than accommodating the moral 'opposition'. Alternatively, the head teacher/governor/parent structure could be given a durable foundation if equipped with guidelines on theory and practice which would enable it to negotiate controversial aspects of the curriculum, and which a nationally agreed programme of school sex education could offer.

Notes

1. In the mid-1980s, Conservative Member of Parliament, James Pawsey led an attack on sex education materials produced for schools by the Brook Advisory Service on the grounds that they were unsuitable for young people. The challenge posed a real threat to the entire government funding for this service, leading to the withdrawal of certain educational pictures.

2. 1944 Education Act

3. op cit. pg 52-3, quoted in Wallis G *Some Ideological Issues in Sex Education in Post-War Britain* unpublished MA dissertation, University of London, Institute of Education, September 1984.

4. Central Advisory Council for Education 1959: '15 to 18' HMSO

5. Newsom Report HMSO 1963

6. *Children and their Primary Schools* HMSO 1967

7. Lukes, S *Power: A Radical View*, Blackwell, London, 1975

8. More recently, it is the DHSS which has taken the initiative on AIDS education, which may extend to schools. It remains to be seen to what extent the future standardisation of a school sex education curriculum will depend upon the need to gain the cooperation of both ministries).

9. Statutory Instruments 1981 No 630 The Education (Schools Information) Regulations DES, HMSO 1981

10. The Responsible Society: *Education or Manipulation: The Ideological and Commercial Exploitation of the Young* 1975

11. ibid.

12. see Responsible Society: *Sex Education in Schools: What Every Parent Should Know* 1982.

PART II:

THE POLITICAL MANAGEMENT OF SCHOOL SEX EDUCATION IN EUROPE

The selective country profiles following aim to compare the British experience of the political management of school sex education with similar processes in: Sweden, Denmark, Federal Republic of Germany, Belgium and Poland. Although the profiles take the similar form of historical and socio-political review, the objective is to highlight in each of these countries developments which may be regarded as valuable to the future organisation of the subject, *nationally* , in Britain.

Chapter 6.1

Sweden: The Evolution of the National Curriculum Handbook

Sweden is exceptional in the field of sex education in many ways. It is of particular relevance to this study that Sweden took the path of national curriculum development of sex education so early, and worked steadily over more than 30 years to provide the means for politicians, teachers and the 'consumers': parents and their children, to understand and where necessary to challenge elements of this curriculum. This was made possible by the creation by successive national commissions of a highly elaborated national curriculum handbook for teachers containing democratically agreed guidelines on philosophy and classroom methodology for all of Sweden.

Historical Background

Sweden has the longest history of 'official' school sex education, and has probably integrated it as an effective learning component of the educational system more successfully than any other country. Its effectiveness can be gauged by a strong reversal of increases in adolescent pregnancies, abortions, and STDs in the 1970s. However, there are historical factors special to Sweden which have assisted in this process.

The country has not been at war since 1814. Such periods of national stress lead to a reinforcement of traditional values to express identity and cohesion. Sweden has, by contrast, been able to discard traditionalism more readily and evolve into a more open society concerning values permitting a long process of social reform.

Secondly, Sweden has been able to avoid the more oppressive heritage of Victorianism on the national consciousness. Industrialisation and urbanisation came late and more gently to this country (end of 19th Century). The effects of the work ethic, factory organisation of labour, austerity and the forms of repression which followed from it did not affect the small population to the extent it did in Britain. In particular, social control over the young weakened rather than increased through the process of urbanisation. Consequently, the society adjusted to the acquired sexual mores of the young much earlier than Britain. Moreover, rural Swedish society had accepted

100

pre-marital sexuality long before, regarding pregnancy as the rite of passage on which marriage had to be based (ie. marriage was then compulsory and expected; the alternative would have been social ostracism).

Thirdly, there was never a significant non-conformist, fundamentalist Christian movement in Sweden as in 19th century England. Moreover the power and influence of the (Lutheran) Church was reduced by its historical alliance with the ruling class, leading to popular resistance to its influence (even though today the Church has 97% allegiance by one of the most secular peoples in the world).

This having been said, the idea that Sweden's history has absolved its population from the strong sex taboos and fear of intimacy which are associated with some other northern European countries would be rejected. Similarly, Jackson's claim,(1) that Sweden has few ethnic and cultural divisions (unlike Britain and the USA) which might undermine its national sex education programme, is questionable. Apart from the fact that modern Sweden is a repository for large numbers of refugees from around the world, one of the very reasons for the creation of a national standardised sex education curriculum was to provide teachers with guidance regarding how pupils with different ethnic values might be 'acculturised' to Swedish (sexual) values without parental misunderstanding or alienation (see below).

Rather, the country is exceptional insofar as it has engaged in a long and systematic public analysis of the psyche of its inhabitants, and the ways in which what are perceived to be negative traits might be corrected through the state educational apparatus, with the assistance of autonomous social movements which included the Swedish Family Planning Association, RFSU. (2)

Contraceptives were first promoted in the 1880s in part due to a fear that an excessive population increase would lead to impoverishment. The traditionalist and progressive dynamic appeared in the form of the Church in confrontation with the labour and women's movements. Through the efforts of charismatic women physicians such as Karolina Widerström, teachers' meetings eventually conceded the need for school sex education. Nevertheless, the first Parliamentary Bill on sex education was rejected. Widerström was responsible for bringing sexuality and reproduction into the public consciousness in a 'respectable' rather than a radical progressive way. She was not a sex reformer, but promoted a medical rationale for sex education to prevent sexually-transmitted disease.

By the 1930s, the Myrdals' famous research of that time identified a resistance to traditional family roles particularly by women, and a resistance to the negative consequences of repeated pregnancy.(3) The corrective to this 'child hostile' mentality took the form of an expansion of state perinatal welfare, free abortion on request and contraceptive counselling for 'family planning' in order to resolve problems of the female reproductive role.(4)

In 1921, the Board of Education accepted, in principle, sex education in secondary but not primary schools. However, only in 1942 did the Government finally recommend (voluntary) education through the local educational authorities. Significantly, this was the result of pressure from a broad spectrum of the public and professions, rather than small reformist pressure groups. The Churches remained resistant until the 1940s.

The Politico-Bureaucratic Management of Sex Education

The administrative structure of the Swedish school system is hierarchic containing four politically-elected agencies, though there is a move to decentralise decision-making to the municipal levels. The *Riksdag* (parliament) stands at the top of the hierarchy, making overriding decisions concerning the goals and general guidelines of the school system, educational legislation, organisation and finance. The government, in the form of the Ministry of Education and Cultural Affairs, takes responsibility for putting its decisions into effect. However, a great deal of implementation is entrusted by the Ministry to the Swedish National Board of Education (Skolöverstyrelsen, SÖ), an executive authority with a politically appointed directorate, the members of which are appointed by the government and represent the political parties in the *Riksdag,* the central employer and employee organisations, municipalities and county councils. The directorate of the National Board has a chair appointed by the government, making the Board relatively independent of the Ministry.

The main tasks of the Board include continuous revision of the curricula, guidelines for research and evaluation, and it is responsible for implementation of the policy decisions of the *Riksdag* and government. Subordinate to the National Board at regional level are the county education boards, also with politically-appointed directorates, assisted by county inspectors of schools. The county boards appoint head teachers and inspect schools to ensure that the policy of the *Riksdag* is being carried out. Local education committees are responsible for the direct political management of schools, which delegate decision-making responsibilities to the head teacher. It is the duty of the head teacher to keep pupils' (school pupil committee) and parents' representatives (PTA) continually *informed*, the latter having the opportunity to offer viewpoints which may influence decision-making. It is the general aim to offer a curriculum of identical range and standard in every school, even though there is scope within the system for variations of method.

Local parental opinion does influence the character of the sex education provided. Teaching materials are produced commercially, although their use is implicitly governed by national guidelines. The Central Board of Social Welfare, historically more progressive, used its influence to counter-balance the more conservative tendencies of the Central Board of Education.

The demand for state school sex education stemmed from concern at the ignorance which was seen to lead to so much marital breakdown, abortion and contraction of STDs in adult life. In response to this, all state schools (there are very few private schools) operate by a nationally standardised curriculum. Part of the credit for the ease by which this component of the school curriculum has been accepted by the majority must come from the *political process* which governed its introduction. While some national decisions in Sweden do not have to depend upon the full democratic process, it was felt that the contentious subject of sex education could only be accepted if subjected to full public scrutiny and participation.

At the heart of the Swedish national programme lies a continuously refined curriculum guide which fulfils the following functions. It has been designed: firstly, as a handbook for classroom practice, secondly, an agenda which permits the subject to be discussed rationally and in an informed way at the various political levels, thirdly, as a detailed advocacy document through which the subject can be communicated and justified to all concerned sections of Swedish society; finally it offers a common agreed foundation for the 'quality control' for teacher training in this field.

Its 'latent function' is to remove as much as possible the 'unknown' from the formal teaching of sexual and personal relationships. A national 'ideological' and practical 'guide to curriculum planning' to resolve differences was devised and refined with the direct involvement of government authority through National Board of Education commissions. The subject was handled therefore through *nationally accepted authorities operating by means of commissions* to resolve policy matters over which social groups customarily differ. Thus, religious influences on the Board led to guidelines in the 1940s which were very conservative. Ironically, their publication assisted the liberal cause as they were dissected by the media. In contrast to Britain, dominant public opinion tended towards accommodation to the 'real' rather than 'ideal'. Thus, moralising was minimised for the sake of guidelines which reflected actual societal values regarding pre-marital sexual behaviour, for example.

Sex education has been included in the school curriculum by Government provision since 1942. The first national guidelines for teachers were published, in a highly concentrated form, in 1945 (70 pages). In 1950, 8 years after the official introduction of (voluntary) school sex education, a questionnaire was sent out to 57 school districts to inquire into the reaction to the guidelines. Twenty-four districts reacted positively, and thirteen negatively. The majority, thirty-one, gave no clear reactions, indicating no strong opposition. However, by 1955, a subsequent investigation revealed that only one county still refused to provide this subject.

Again the guidelines were revised and expanded to take objections into account. A subsequent refined and elaborated version (240 pages) was issued in 1956. This publication was enormously successful and influential among Swedish teachers (88% of a survey of teachers - mostly form-masters and biology teachers reporting having consulted it in their work).

Through this process of national commission, consultation and refinement, the government eventually felt it had a mandate to make the subject compulsory in 1956, even though this was hardly necessary considering that very few schools were still not teaching the subject voluntarily, according to the guidelines. However, it was recognised that there existed a difference between 'official acceptance' and 'real implementation', which legal obligation could correct. Certain sections of the public remained dissatisfied with elements of the content and rationale. The government response to this was to establish a national commission to review the subject in 1964. These criticisms were seriously considered, resulting in a small shift of emphasis. The 1964 Commission proposed that sex education should start at the pre-school level, when children are three to six years old, and continue through the higher levels. There should also be collaboration between the home and school concerning methods of presenting the subject, the content having been established.

Only by 1970, could the government be sure that every young person was exposed to some form of sex education. Before 1960, the content and quality of sex education actually provided and absorbed was unknown. This led to large scale government funding for national research into Swedish sexual behaviour and the influence of sex education. The Swedish 'Kinsey Report', Zetterberg's *On Sexual Life in Sweden* was published in 1969. It focused upon teaching in primary schools during the first six years. This was accompanied by a special public report on what the teachers thought of sex education teaching. A further study *by subject* was undertaken for classes 7,8,9. Due to a feeling that teachers would probably overstate the quality of the teaching they were giving, a survey of pupil opinion was also undertaken. The results revealed a remarkable symmetry between the attitudes of the teachers and those of the pupils. A large minority reported that sex education was neither 'good' nor 'bad'.

A fourth version of the curriculum guide was introduced in 1974, containing a revised programme concerning content and working methods, largely as a result of the increased openness towards sexuality. This method of nationally organised and legitimised cycle of: research, authorship, consultation, and revision has continued exhaustively. The revised draft 1974 guidelines, which received official endorsement and were finally published in 1977, were first submitted for scrutiny by 60 bodies and experts. The 1977 *Instruction Concerning Interpersonal Relations* represents the most comprehensive and sophisticated approach to the subject in any country. (A full English translation of this work of 300 pages was produced in 1981).

The Evolving Rationale for Swedish Sex Education

The pervasive social welfare system in Sweden has provided the impetus for a national, standardised assault, through the education process, on problems of adolescent physical and psychological health in sexual matters. However, there is a long tradition of *value-neutrality* in Swedish schools, (which originated in resistance to conveying the values of the state Church at the exclusion of others such as atheistic socialism). As a result, schools have been perceived as institutions whose task was to convey factual knowledge rather than moral values, the latter left to the home.

This profoundly influenced (and helped resolve some problems of) the first official sex education guidelines. School sex education, as understood in the late 1950s and early 1960s concerned preparation for sexual life in the form of instruction in physiology, reproduction and contraception. This instruction was based on the desire to remove the consequences of simple ignorance of, and taboos connected with, the working of one's own and one's partner's body in order to avoid any physiological and psychosexual problems in later life, or put another way to enjoy one's sexual life fully. Sexuality has always been perceived as a (potentially) positive force for pleasure and human intimacy.

The libertarian philosophy in Swedish social policy of the 1960s and 1970s so perceived sexuality as a private and positive force that legal constraints on sexual expression in the media were removed. What was not anticipated however was the extent to which commercial interests made use of these developments to encourage the very sexual depravity (pornography) which liberal policy makers had hoped would be eliminated.

A consequent shift of approach is reflected strongly in the revisions of the official guidelines on school sex education in the 1970s, when it was conceived (partly in response to public opinion) that schools should not and could not evade the responsibility of conveying fundamental moral values to their pupils. Thus, the commission which created the 1974 and 1977 versions of the handbook concluded by recommending that greater stress be placed on the significance of personal relationships 'facts' in addition to the explaining about the technical-physical aspects of sexuality.

They went further than accommodating objections to the earlier guidelines but took into account the contemporary changes in Swedish life, noting that the school reflected the traditionalistic influence of many who believed sex education belonged in the home, that pre-marital sex should never be condoned and that information about sexuality encouraged promiscuity. A minority of physicians and religious individuals had petitioned the government for a stricter approach to sexual norms in teaching. The commission felt that this did not reflect the reality in which young people lived and it was rejected. Pointing out that many parents did not object to teenage sons and daughters having steady relations including sexual relations if acting responsibly, it was argued:

'It would be wrong in principle and fatal to teaching if the school were morally to reject these young people and their parents. The attitude of the school cannot be decided by reference to a majority'(5)

The 1977 Curriculum Guide: 'Instruction Concerning Interpersonal Relations' (6)

The title denotes that the narrow term 'sex education' to describe the content of the guide is misleading, referring instead to 'interpersonal relations' (though there is disagreement over the value of using the English word 'instruction'. It contains the following components:

1.   A full sociological-philosophical-moral **justification** for the programme (to the parent, politician etc.) in the form of : goals, directions, commentaries on the main focus for the teacher to pursue. This includes a methodology for the management of value issues *vis-à-vis* facts which avoids the stance of value relativism.

2.   Directions on **working method**: strategies of handling difficult subjects in the classroom - a code of practice both for teacher and pupil.

3.   Elaboration of means of dealing with **controversies in teaching** (with philosophical/ rational justifications). For example: homosexuality, the teaching of ethnic minorities.

4.   A **compendium of facts** (knowledge base) designed to furnish the teacher with an overview of the fields relevant to the subject. Where actual information is not included, references are offered. The import of the compendium is that the teacher should not have to delve much deeper into

any single subject via commercial publications in order to satisfy classroom demands. This large section of the guide contains information on anatomy, physiology, differing philosophies of life, social and psychological issues and relevant legislation. Thus, it is not presumed that school teachers are in a position to locate and interpret all pertinent information themselves.

The following presents extracts of the guide in order to convey the flavour of the detail with which the Commission addresses the teacher, parent and public reader. It should be noted that content and method are reviewed according to three age ranges: junior (7-10 years), intermediate (10-12 years), and senior (13-16 years). The guide sets out the following as the general goals of the *school* (*vis-à-vis* any other agent):

A. 'They are to acquire a knowledge of anatomy, physiology, psychology, ethics, and social relations calculated to improve their prospects of achieving interpersonal relations characterised by responsibility, consideration and care for their fellow beings, and in this way experiencing sexuality as a source of happiness together with another person. This has five components:

a) *Promotion of the capacity for intimacy.* This is seen as a prerequisite for sexual life as a source of happiness. It is noted that sexuality can take place without intimacy, but with intimacy, sexuality satisfies a profound human need. But this is not designated a precondition of decent human existence (ie. one can remain non-sexually active and be fully human); nor is this goal an absolute. It does not suggest that it is morally-inferior to have shorter-term relationships; nor should it be over-idealised.

b) *Preparation for family life.* This refers to the contribution of families to social cohesion etc., though the guide does not restrict the definition to a nuclear arrangement. It must be explained that there are variations of family structure (which may be equally good), and that divorce is sometimes necessary. (Definition: 'Any type of relationship between a man, woman, or child, or any two of these parties, which is characterised by the intention of permanent association and the assumption of responsibility.'(7)

c) *Preparation for social and sexual relationships* in adolescence. It is felt that young people should not be left alone in the difficult task of framing their own norms and lifestyles.

d) *Prevention of STDs and unwanted pregnancy.*

e) *Impact of social and cultural conditions on quality of relationships* (stresses of working conditions, housing). It is important here to broaden the perspective beyond Sweden/Europe to include the pros/cons of interpersonal relations in other cultures or social systems.

It is intended that these objectives remove the danger of sexuality being seen as something separate from society, though this must not obscure 'the (probable) existence of universal and timeless individual-psychological experience of love and sexuality.' (8) Moreover, 'sexuality should be viewed as a positive aspect of life'.

B. 'They are to acquire a knowledge of beliefs and ideologies and of values concerning sexual and other interpersonal relations, so as to be able to accept basic (common) values which the curriculum states are to be highlighted and encouraged, and so as to be able to adopt standpoints concerning divergent values which the curriculum states are to be presented objectively and impartially.'(9)

Recognising that individuals differ in their moral interpretation of sexual behaviour, the guide confronts the problem head on, rather than delegating the problem to individual teachers to enter the contentious area alone. In the past the teacher was expected to restrict the school's contribution to this education by providing factual information in a value-neutral way. On this basis, the pupil was left to acquire his/her own value system (through the influence of parents, friends etc). Recognising the weaknesses of this approach to the subject (the potential danger of provision of objective information to young people without the means to interpret it responsibly), the current guide provides a way of adjudicating over what constitutes an acceptable standard of sexual morality. It distinguishes between 'basic' or 'common' societal values over which there would be little dispute, and controversial values. This is to say that it does not take for granted that society operates more or less according to a code of values but makes them explicit.

Concerning fundamental societal values . The guide reminds the reader that, 'Contrary to what many people suppose, there is an extensive community of values in this field. There are a number of important points on which, instead of wrestling with divergent values, one can therefore assert, without infringing anybody's liberties, that certain things are right and proper'. It also warns the teacher however not to let discussion of values dominate teaching.

Examples . The following values are proposed to be encouraged: 'democratic principles of tolerance, partnership and equality of rights'... 'respect for truth and justice, for the dignity of man, for the inviolability of human life... for the right of personal privacy.'(10)

Respect for the 'dignity of man' is to be used as a means of reminding the class that nobody can be allowed to regard another person merely as a means of catering for his/her own interests and needs; and that causing an unwanted pregnancy is a serious manifestation of this. The discussion of the value opens the way for provision of information and instruction of a medical nature though, for example: 'gonorrhoea and its avoidance should not be treated solely as a medical and technical problem', when exposing a person to risk of infection contravenes the fundamental value.

Respect for the right of personal privacy is to be interpreted to raise the problem of male (sexual) assault on women, against which acts schools must 'mobilise opinion'. It also includes a rejection of pornography, meaning the use of persons as 'objects' of sexual gratification, rather than individuals.

Respect for equality of rights implies rejection of racial discrimination and discrimination against homosexuals. Tolerance is to be nurtured, except in relation to values and behaviour which are contrary to what the Curriculum terms basic and common values (eg. prohibition of sexual/physical cruelty).

Concerning classroom practice in respect of fundamental values. 'The purpose of instruction is then to elucidate what the pupils in many cases have already vaguely sensed. To this end the teacher can adopt two distinct courses. (Firstly) 'He can say with conviction that one kind of behaviour is obviously right and the other wrong... Strong emotional commitment here on the teacher's part can help young persons to deepen and consolidate their own values'; (secondly) 'The situation where basic values are subjected to free scrutiny (with the recognition that these values uphold the foundations of society)... There is an important psychological reason for using this method. It is the only way in which a person's values can become a manifestation of his or her individual lifestyle'.

This represents a rejection by the Swedish commission of the authoritarian-psychological aversion method of teaching values.

Concerning controversial values relating to sexuality: The guide offers the following comments on this category of values. 'The school systems of democratic countries have to try to remain neutral concerning divergent values in society... eg. schools must not be used for party political propaganda' (11); therefore, 'Instruction must be objective, ie. factual and impartial... impartiality is particularly vital when dealing with beliefs and ideologies, values and controversial viewpoints generally. In situations of this kind it is essential for different views to be balanced against one another...*unless the democratically defined goals and guidelines of the Curriculum state explicitly that certain values are to be presented and encouraged* (our emphasis). The mode of presentation must not be such that the teacher identifies with or rejects the controversial views that are being dealt with. Of course, this does not prevent the teacher from stating his personal views.'

'Whereas instruction concerning basic and common values is evaluative and intended to exert influence, instruction concerning differing values is objective...All parents must be able to send their children to school with equal confidence, in the assurance that the school will not influence them in favour of one or other of the rival views and beliefs....The Upper Secondary School Curriculum includes a detailed presentation of the values to be presented and encouraged, but at the same time it affirms *that it should always be left to the pupil to accept or reject a value on the strength of his own independent judgement* (our emphasis).Where instruction on the subject of common values is concerned... the teacher must point out such values and stand up for them, while at the same time making it clear by his attitude that the ultimate decision rests with the pupil.' (12)

(Alternatively)... the teacher does not indicate any standpoint on the part of society or the school system. He simply tries to explain the nature of the differing values and their implications. The pupil is still faced with the task of thinking for himself, and making his own decision. In this sense, both types of instruction are objective.

The teacher is expected to endorse sexual fidelity within a regular relationship as a fundamental Swedish value, explaining its full (psychological) meaning in the sense of human need for common identity. However, in terms of facts, it is also necessary to reveal that this is an area of *differing values,* as some regard permanent fidelity as God-given; others that it is desirable, socially/psychologically; others that it is unnecessary and unrealistic to desire such fidelity:

'The mode of presentation must not be such that a teacher identifies with or rejects the controversial views that are being dealt with. Of course, this does not prevent the teacher from stating his personal views.' (13)

(Where the teacher makes personal opinion) 'A demand of this kind from the pupils can be regarded as a positive feature of the teaching situation, but the teacher is not under any obligation to state his personal views on questions of values.' (14)

Examples (from teaching at the middle level). On the subject of homosexuality:

'There is often a great deal of prejudice and contempt among boys in their early teens concerning homosexuality. For this reason it should be made clear that confirmed homosexuality is deeply rooted

110

in the personality of the individual concerned...Discrimination should be rejected as other forms of discrimination are... Homosexuals should feel that they are free to organise their mutual relations as they themselves wish... During this period a young person may feel attracted to a person of the same sex. This reaction is usually transitory. Young persons should be informed that impulses of this kind do not as a rule betoken homosexuality.'(15)

On the subject of contraception:

'It must be pointed out that the use of contraceptives conflicts with certain people's religious and ethical convictions and that these convictions are to be respected. It is not the business of schools to try to inculcate other attitudes.'

On the subject of abortion:

The facts about the abortion law are to be explained; in particular, that every woman has a legal right to decide if she wishes to give birth to a child or not. The abortion issue is one on which opinion is deeply divided. Thus, 'It is very important in school instruction to avoid adopting a standpoint for or against any of the main ethical views concerning this question.'

Of family life:

'Although young people do not regard the formation of a family as something imminent, schools should focus their thoughts on this reality. There is one thing *which the great majority have in common in this connection,* and on which teaching can be based, namely the conviction that marriage (or its counterpart) requires fidelity. There are those who feel that this is a prejudice, but this does not alter the fact that the great majority advocate fidelity (based on surveys of the young as well as adults)...(in addition) ' the Christian view of marriage should be presented with particular emphasis on points which different denominations have in common'....Another large group has partly abandoned this view, regarding marriage, whether by religious or civil ceremony, as the introduction to a sincere effort to found a lasting family. but at the same time to dissolve it if the strains become excessive.'(16)

Background Knowledge for Teachers

The Manual refers to the 'sexual instinct' (17) within a brief discussion of theories of sexuality (viz: the impact of Freud). It also offers an historical dimension, and contemporary survey data on (Swedish) sexual behaviour. On the question of factual instruction on matters of sexual mores the guide recommends that:

> 'the presentation may only include statements *which are judged to be true or which are highly probable. If, for special reasons, statements are presented which are judged to be of limited probability, this should be made clear*. School instruction should be based on available research findings on this subject. The 'impartiality principle' can be difficult to live up to...it should be made clear to pupils that objectivity in the absolute sense is unattainable when dealing with differing values....the teacher is not under any obligation (from school or pupils) to state his personal view on questions of values.' (our emphasis)

The guide accedes that fears have been expressed that teaching of this kind may give rise to a moral relativism on the part of pupils; that one cannot arrive at a set opinion concerning right and wrong because there are issues on which the school does not express an opinion. However, 'the task of schools is not to inculcate a relativistic attitude but to contribute towards a deeper and better motivated conviction involving a greater degree of personal commitment....One may also say that schools must be neutral towards differing values in order to avoid infringing the right of the family, voluntary organisations and religious denominations to campaign for their views.' (18)

The commission also recommends that teaching should utilise the factual knowledge available of standards and behaviour in the field of personal relationships, allowing the teacher to correct widely held misconceptions concerning the sexual habits of young people:

> 'One specific cause of misconceptions concerning the sexual habits of young people is the predilection of certain "liberal-minded" mass media to select and interview promiscuous young people and present them as typical. This is another reason for giving a more realistic picture. It is also necessary, if he or she is to avoid two erroneous premises in teaching, namely that all of the older students have had intercourse, or that practically none of them have.'(19)

Examples of Managing Classroom Issues

Guidance for the teacher is offered regarding common classroom problems, on the premise that there is a 'need to construct a secure environment in school, so that both adults and pupils will feel free to express their feelings, thoughts and opinions.'(20)

'Matters will be raised in a natural manner if instruction is essentially based on the children's spontaneous questions and choices of topics': (21)

'This also means that teaching must deal with the question of sexual debuts occurring before the debutants are mentally capable of coping with a sexual relationship. Early contacts of this kind also involve a greater risk of inability to take consistent precautions against unwanted pregnancy and venereal infection. Schools should make active efforts to prevent young persons from getting into situations of this kind... (nevertheless)... teaching must be designed so as to cater both for those young persons who have not embarked on sexual relations - and who in many cases do not wish to do so until later in life - and for those who have entered into such relations. Both groups of young persons must feel that their situation is being taken seriously and that every attitude involving responsibility and consideration is respected.' (22)

'The human attitudes and living patterns of children and teenagers evolve through a process of interaction with others. For this reason, instruction concerning interpersonal relations cannot be confined to individual lessons or working periods... (but) form a natural ingredient of work in many subjects throughout the pupils' school careers.' (23)

On the question of the vocabulary of this education:

'Young people... often acquire an insecure attitude toward sexuality... The teacher should deal with serious questions, problems and conjectures... even if the pupils seem to phrase them... in a manner which the teacher finds offensive... Pupils should be able to use words and phrases which they have learned and whose meaning is known to everybody. But it must be considered equally natural for the teacher to avoid expressions which he knows are liable to offend some young persons and adults for one reason or another..the teacher must set an example concerning language... help to establish a usage based on commonly accepted words and expressions... it is important for pupils to grow accustomed to talking about sex and interpersonal relations, but it is equally imperative to avoid ever forcing a person to take part in a discussion or to declare his or her values.' (24)

Of teaching aids:

'As regards illustrations in aids for sexual relations, the Commission proposes that the following guidelines be applied. In the case of anatomical and physiological illustrations of the scientific type, no principles of selection need to be applied other than consideration to the pupil's capacity for comprehension and motivation at the level in question. No factual knowledge in these fields is unsuitable or injurious.'

Aspects of the Consultation Procedure

In recognition of the most effective ways of allaying parental anxieties and possible prejudices, the guide expressedly states that first and foremost the basic principles underlying this instruction should be presented to parents. Only then should the actual content of the instruction be discussed:

'Instruction concerning interpersonal relations is to be planned by the school management in cooperation with a working party...the part will vary by school according to composition of staff but will include the main teaching staff, other teachers with an interest in the field; the school doctor, nurse, welfare officer, school psychologist; an outside expert: midwife, gynaecologist, priest, etc.'

'Instruction Concerning Interpersonal Relations calls for cooperation between school staff and parents. The children's security is greatly dependent on a form of contact between school and parents which provides opportunities of discussion and mutual influence. Parents must be told how the teacher intends talking to their children..teachers for their part should be informed of parental views concerning sex education.'

The Problem of Ethnic and National Minorities

One central *raison d'être* of the Swedish curriculum guide is to confront the problem of implementing a nationally-standardised programme of school sex education in a way which does not exclude or produce resistance in ethnic, cultural or religious minorities. This question, which is a major ethical and practical impediment to standardised sex education in any educational system, takes up a significant part of the handbook. An elaborate and persuasive rationale for a single sex education for all social groups is presented not only as a feasible but socially-necessary undertaking. The justification is aimed to assist the teacher in the classroom content and as an 'official' (governmental) statement to the consumer.

The Minority Situation: 'If there are several different ethnic groups in a society, efforts can be made to find either a pluralistic or a monistic solution to the problem of interpersonal relations. ...A fully implemented pluralistic solution requires the ethnic group to be large and internally united so that they will be viable communities in their own right at the same time as they participate actively in the majority community..they can retain their ethnic, cultural and linguistic identity...In a monistic society, on the other hand, a distinct majority-minority situation prevails which has become acute and controversial as a result of immigration. The majority may comprise 95 per cent of the population. Its language, culture, social organisation and political decisions permeate practically the whole of society...The minorities will spend most of their lives in the world of the majority - for example as regards working conditions, social customs, language and values..The members of a minority are bound to experience a world created by the majority...(25)

Swedish society endeavours to neutralise the discriminatory effect of minority status of immigrants (language learning facility; social benefits etc). On the subject of potential clash of values, it recognises that power is vested in the majority community. This being so, how can majority position be upheld while retaining respect for that of the minority.

The family and sexual morals are only one of the fields in which some immigrants are subjected to a painful confrontation, but it is probably the field which most profoundly affects their personalities. The guide provides illustrations of differences in the values of typical immigrant communities and the host society (eg. around the role and status of women). The commentary concludes:

'As a result some ethnic groups experience the instruction received by their children in accordance with Swedish curricula as an encroachment on areas in which the family rejects all influence from the norms and values of the majority community. On one hand they emphasise the right to privacy; on the other no pupil may be excluded from instruction concerning sexual and interpersonal relations... Every growing person must be considered entitled to receive competent and considerate instruction concerning sexual matters.'

This is justified on the grounds that the young person will be exposed to a variety of competing images of Swedish society through the free media, which, without school education offering a factual and moral basis for judgement, would lead to confusion and misunderstandings which could be injurious both to the youth and members of the society with whom he/she must relate. This is particularly acute in the realm of sexual and interpersonal relations. Compulsory sex education in this respect is defended on the grounds of moral protection of the youth from the society, and society from the youth.

The differentiation of fundamental and controversial values discussed above is critical here:

'...schools should be at pains to inform parents that sex education must be based on respect for different values. Parents should be able to count on their basic ethical views in this context being accurately and respectfully presented... It may also be appropriate for schools to inform parents of the main outlines of sex education...The discussion in class of differences between majority and minority groups and of their respective values can lead to fruitful cultural exchange...'

There is one field, however, in which cultural conflict cannot be prevented, namely the fundamental view taken concerning the relationship between a man and a woman. This is one of the fields in which school instruction is not meant to be objective in the sense of neutral. On the contrary, schools are obliged to communicate these fundamental values to all pupils:

'(Goals and guidelines of the Swedish Parliament: "Schools should work for the promotion of equality between men and women- in the family, labour market and elsewhere in society".)...To this end...girls and boys should work together in groups on similar tasks....These directions mean that some immigrant pupils will encounter an explicit, negative valuation of the attitude toward the domestic and social tasks of men and women which are taken for granted in their families.'

In sum, Swedish schools must continue to work towards greater equality between the sexes as a fundamental societal value, even if this differs from those of minority groups. The compulsory school curriculum stipulates respect for the distinctive characteristics of other peoples... at the same time enunciating and maintaining the values of the Swedish school system, adopting the attitude that each individual is ultimately responsible for the standpoint he chooses. Not even values of fundamental importance in Swedish society are to be presented in authoritarian terms:

'The really important thing in this context is for the younger generation to be able to ask vital contemporary questions about people's personal and social problems.'... 'Sex education itself implies a cultural conflict..traditional silence on sexual matters... This silence plays a vital part in their child education and is a means of upholding sexual discipline generally... Although sex education in Sweden does not adopt a particular standpoint concerning the choice between restrictive or more permissive sexual morality, this still leaves the minorities concerned with a problem. The objective line taken on this subject in the classroom provides parents with an assurance that their children will not be subjected to an authoritative conditioning in favour of a different opinion from that espoused by their parents, but the factual information supplied concerning anatomy and physiology... nonetheless amounts to a transmission of knowledge (contrary to values of parents).'(26)

Nevertheless, such parents cannot be permitted to withdraw children from such classes:

'This is not an acceptable solution...(for) every day they see numerous expressions of sexual frankness... pictures, articles in press, radio and television... It is not true to say that these children and young persons lead secluded lives dominated by the values and attitudes of their own ethnic group, and that Swedish sex education shatters the calm, creating a cultural conflict which could otherwise be avoided. The cultural conflict is there already...This being so there is a need for the qualitatively superior information concerning facts and values, coupled with evaluative conditioning, which good sex education can supply.'

'It seems likely that even parents tormented by this situation could be convinced by the following argument to the effect that pupils would suffer greater harm as a result of non-participation (because of such young persons being excluded from the conversations of their peers). Also mentioned are the question of integrated curriculum and the problem of reaction from other pupils to absence of minority.'

Conclusions

No society can avoid the process of erecting the structures necessary to deal with school sex education. Moreover, all the countries reviewed, although different in the time they have come to deal with this and to some extent the manner (suited to their wider political system) have come to deal with the same requirements. There are a number of paths to fulfilling these requirements.

Sex educators need the moral support of 'official' guidelines which address all contentious areas. Such a legitimation cannot be sought in the commercial market of sex education texts. The chairman of the 1977 National Commission has noted:

'It was the official guidelines in the handbooks of 1945 and 1956 which deeply influenced Swedish sex education when it was still in formation. They gave the teachers courage to start something so shocking as sex education. They got official support through a programme edited by the Central Board of Schools. (Consequently) it became impossible to attack the teachers for giving this education...The handbook gave them a distinct form of pedagogical presentation, pointed out the necessary items, gave the teachers fundamental knowledge and discussed the methodological problems.'(27)

The challenge is familiar - to minimise, through national government interference, the impasse and factionalism created by traditionalist and progressive forces. This would eventually be resolved by minimising traditionalism not through ignoring or alienation but by a level of accommodation.

It is insufficient to resolve problems of content without the political means to permit public involvement. The outstanding feature of Sweden's history of school sex education is the enormous lengths which official commissions have gone to to publicly air areas of potential controversy and elaborately *justify* the formulas adopted. This must include government in a capacity in which it is an interested party among others and will submit to authority of a Commission. This Commission is representative and respected. Consequently, as has been shown, it does not exist just to deliver the judgement of the majority in society but a rational balancing of all positions including the reality of behaviour in society.

A secondary essential component is the elaboration of an agenda for teaching in such a form that everyone in the society can have access to it: the handbook, which does not just set out the content and working methods to be used in the classroom but the rationale for practice. Each version has helped substantially to *form* the pattern of all sex education. In so doing it informs the public precisely what the school will and will not provide in this area. The handbook is a direct effect (reflection) of a hierarchical and consultative political management structure which has managed to remain free from *party political interference.*

But at present it is believed that the handbook is only systematically used by the most enthusiastic and progressive educators in colleges and in-service training and is little consulted by the bulk of teachers, themselves (while 60,000 teachers have sex education in their curriculum, only 20,000 copies of the handbook have been sold). Moreover, teacher training in sex education is provided on a very small scale, and where it is provided it is unpopular (although some in-service training has a good reputation). In 1978, three-day courses in interpersonal relations were introduced by the National Board of Education because of fears about rising teenage pregnancy. These courses were discontinued because of lack of take-up. Teachers were simply not interested in a formal learning approach to this subject for themselves, no more would they propose such an approach for their pupils.

Investigations have revealed that practically all pupils receive and are satisfied with sex education, even though the quantity and quality is found to vary (it is least developed at the nursery school level). In practice, teachers use the range of subjects in the curriculum to discuss issues of sexuality, deciding the content of the sex education he/she provides according to the accepted approaches. (28)

Notes

1. Jackson, S *Sexuality and Childhood* Blackwell, Oxford 1982 pg 192

2. Riksforbundet for Sexuell Upplysning; literally: Swedish Association for Sex Education. For its historical emergence see: RFSU *Vision, Reality, Activities* PO Box 17006, S-104 62 Stockholm 1981

3. Myrdal, A and G *Crisis and Population* 1934 (English version: Myrdal, *A Nation and Family* 1941) MIT Press (Cambridge 1968)

4. This concern has continued to the present. In 1968, Sweden became the first country to frame a government policy of achieving equality between the sexes. All legislation and policy must be directed to replacing the male breadwinner, female homemaker roles with a partnership of independent individuals.

5. USSU *Sexual och Samlevnadsandervisning* Utbildningsdepartementet 1974 (English summary).

6. National Swedish Board of Education *Instruction Concerning Interpersonal Relations* Liber Utbildningsforlaget Stockholm 1981

7. ibid. pg 12

8. ibid. pg 15

9. ibid. pg 10

10. ibid. pg 16

11. ibid. pg 15

12. ibid. pg 22

13. ibid. pg 13

14. ibid. pg 23

15. ibid. pg 58

16. ibid. pg 83
17. ibid. pg 31
18. ibid. pg 24
19. USSU 1974 op cit.
20. National Swedish Board of Education 1981 op cit. pg36
21. ibid. pg 12
22. ibid. pg 28
23. ibid. pg 36
24. ibid. pg 36
25. ibid. pg 109
26. ibid. pg 118
27. Personal communication with Carl-Gustav Boëthius.
28. Investigations of effects of sex education on the sexual debut began in 1986. It has been discovered that young girls are resisting boys' requests for first intercourse more strongly (increased by 1 year since 1960s). It is also discovered that the year of first intercourse has been reversed (now girls have their sexual debut one year earlier than boys). This indicates that the 'double standard' has been undermined by education. There is also a levelling- off of the period of menarche and sexual initiation. In addition there has been a 40% decrease in gonorrhoea in 5 years (leaving the fight against the more recent clamydia to be continued).

Chapter 6.2

Denmark: Regulating Classroom Interaction

The detail with which the Danish state has addressed the issue of sex education practice compares almost with Sweden, though the emphasis is different. In Denmark, greater attention has been paid to rules of conduct between teacher and pupil rather than the content of this dialogue. This reflects some anxiety to ensure that the rights and responsibilities of teacher, school, physician, and pupil remain clear in order to maintain confidence in the system.

Historical Background

As in the case of Sweden, Denmark also emerged without the full impact which the Christian tradition had on sexual mores in the cultures of other parts of Europe. For example, rural Denmark also tolerated adolescent pre-marital sexual relations, pregnancy being the rite of passage into marriage. While 'Victorian' attitudes to sex did harden during the 19th century, they appear to have had more effect on the legal superstructure of the Danish state, than on its culture.

The perceived need for sex education by those in the teaching, medical and caring professions (which included early feminists), was in part a consequence of the increasingly repressive attitude to sexuality which appeared in the 19th century. The Danish movement for sexual reform was touched by developments in feminist politics and medical-psychological sexology. However that stream which evolved into the Danish family planning movement also held to a more romantic ideal of the total person who must be protected from the societal corruption by education. E. Hoffmeyer, the most important theoretician of what would become Danish sex education, professed a humanistic belief in the need to integrate bodily with social harmony, sexuality being a vital *positive* component in this equation. However, socio-economic forces threatened to pervert this human 'wholeness' and integration, resulting in inhibitions and repression. In modern urban-industrial society, these forces must be counteracted by formal sex education.(1)

This conception of the importance of avoiding sexual repression was central to the philosophy of the Danish Family Planning Association, whose members had an important influence on the early national commissions on the subject.(2) Although Freud is not held up as a formative influence on the Association's thinking, founder president Agnete Braestrup's writings do reflect a child psychology which is essentially Freudian: that for the well-being of children in later life it is important that they do not develop mental 'blocks' to sexual matters because of the devious or ignorant answers offered by parents and other adults, which would be so difficult to remove in later life.

Doubtless influenced by the Danish sex reform movement, progressive school teachers, particularly in the capital, had been covertly giving their own kind of sex education to pupils as early as the 1930s, when such instruction was still illegal. This was done out of a perception of need for such knowledge, due partly to the fact that in the Danish school system, the form teacher remains with the same pupils throughout their primary and secondary education.

Thus, sex education was advanced through the efforts of the enlightened Copenhagen medical and educational professional classes in the years leading up to 1946. Other factors influenced this development: in particular, the feminist movement and the first population commission. After World War 1 women entered factory work, female employment creating a desire for smaller families through the use of contraceptive methods. This impetus for change in family size was encouraged by the government. For in the 1930s there had been a National Population Commission (*Betænkning: Befolningskommission)* which reported on the economic threat posed by too fast an increase in population. It also covered the area of sexual hygiene and education and recommended that contraceptive education be given to the young, despite it being illegal at that time.

The efforts of the sex reformers so impressed a sympathetic Director of Education in the Copenhagen municipality that the local education authority commissioned the first pedagogy of sex education *(Undervisningen: Seksualbelræing* Københavns Kommunale Skoleveksen 1946). He was, however, unable to persuade the government to take similar steps for the whole of Denmark.

Rather, it was the Swedish national commission on sex education which first reported in the 1950s, which was to spur the Danish government to inaugurate a similar commission at the beginning of the 1960s, due to increasing public concern about the numbers of unwanted pregnancies particularly among adolescents. The Ministry of Education eventually conceded that state school sex education was essential, acting on this by making adjustments to the school curriculum guidelines of the day (*Vejledning Seksualundervisning i Folkeskolen* : Guide to the Teaching of Sex Education in Public Schools).

Another significant historical development at this time was the publication of a thesis on women's sexual behaviour by psychiatrist, Kirsten Auken in 1953. This was based on a sample of 315 women born between 1910-27, and revealed that only 3.5% reported receiving any education about sexuality.

Irrespective of these events, school sex education is believed to have become widespread by the 1950s due to the initiative taken by school teachers, themselves. To this day, the form teacher takes responsibility for such education (in collaboration with the school nurse or physician), the visiting 'expert' sex educator being alien to the long term teacher-pupil relationship fostered by the system.

Due to the influence particularly of the Danish National Women's Council and the 'Motherhelp' movement, in 1961, a commission on sex education was set up by the Prime Minister, himself. The resulting 1968 report, *Seksualundervisning i Folkeskole*n (Sex Education in Primary Schools) recommended that sex education be given throughout the 'Folkeskolen' (state school) system as an integrated part of compulsory subjects. There was no obligation for teachers to undertake this subject. The report was based on the idea that sexual instruction be adapted to children's differing degrees of maturity but that it should not be perceived as a special field of learning or 'speculation'. If it was to be dealt with in the classroom in a spontaneous manner, it followed that it must be integrated with other subjects.

In 1966 the Public Hygiene Act integrated family planning into the Danish national health service, giving young people the right to consult physicians without parental knowledge on the subject, the first in the world to award this right.

A 1970 proposed amendment to the *State Schools Act* proposed to extend this provision to primary schools, and that the subject should henceforth be compulsory, due to concern about the effectiveness of voluntary teaching. Moreover, with the assent of the National Teacher's Association, school boards, parents' associations, and the National Association of Municipal Councils, teachers were no longer to be permitted to avoid this teaching. Integrated instruction was to be accompanied by special discrete classes on sex education in the 6th and 9th years.

Within the limits of the law, schools nevertheless have a say in what is taught and how this is taught. Moreover, the state felt it necessary to commission the Curriculum Committee to create new guidelines for curriculum design and practice to replace those of 1961 and to cater for the new regulations.

The 1970 Act was not passed without media debate, this revealing a widespread concern over consequences for sexual morality and creating objections from religious individuals (though not official groups or denominational). However, this still did not add up to the kind of resistance that might have been expected in other European countries. It had the full support of the medical and teaching professions, and was based on the 1968 report of the sex education commission. Moreover, the media played a highly responsible role in adjudicating on this issue, largely as a result of its traditional anti-Church sympathies.

In 1971 the most extensive guidelines yet created for teachers were published *(Vejledning om Seksualoplysning i Folkeskolen* : Guidance on Sexual Orientation in Primary Schools) (see below).

In 1972, partly as a result of second thoughts by the Teachers Association and as a result of the case before the European Court of Human Rights (see below), the 1970 Act was amended due to an intervention by the Minister of Education. This amendment permitted teachers to opt out of the specific (ie. un-integrated) sex education teaching to be given in the 6th and 9th years. Parents would also be given the option to withdraw their children from these specific classes.

In the period since the 1971 Education Act, there has been a general Law on Education (1975) which revised all subjects, leading to a new commission (currently in progress) to specifically examine the working of the guidelines on sex education. Thus, in 1976, the subject of 'health education' became more clearly defined and placed in the curriculum. This raises the need to better integrate sex and health education into one subject.

In 1986, the Minister of Education appointed a further National Commission to review the progress made on the basis of the 1971-2 guidelines, and to update them in the light of changing social values and circumstances such as the arrival of AIDS. This Commission has nine members, six appointed for their specialist knowledge of sex education work: school physician, school psychologist, nurses and teachers; a representative of the Danish Teachers Association, Danish Nurses Organisation and the Council for Preventive Health.

Political-bureaucratic Structure

In contrast to its neighbour Sweden, with its highly centralised social welfare administration, Denmark has an extensively de-centralised political-administrative system, in which all domestic decision-making is dealt with at the commune level. In the educational sphere this extends to the participation of parents groups in decision-making about the curriculum and running of the school.

The 'Folkeskole' is the responsibility of the local authority both in respect of curriculum and administration. The Ministry of Education concerns itself with the content of only a certain type of school education to be deemed compulsory. However, it can only make 'suggestions' for the curriculum proper. These compulsory subjects are to be integrated throughout the curriculum and must include: health/ sex education; road safety; comparative religion and Swedish/ Norwegian. Nevertheless, nowadays the Ministry of Education actively promotes sex education particularly through teachers' organisations.

State schools are run by the municipal councils, the highest education authority in each of some 275 municipalities in that country, as well as by a school commission and a school board.

It should be stressed that the local authority is totally responsible for the 'Folkeskole'. There is a centrally elaborated curriculum in primary and secondary schools and in institutions for training teachers. However, the national law merely prescribes the general fields of education which must be covered.

The *school commission* (skolekommissionen) is as a general rule composed of eleven members of whom six are elected by the municipal council and five by the parents. The commission, in consultation with the teachers' council and within the limits laid down by law, prepares the curriculum of the schools within its district. The curriculum must be approved by the municipal council. To assist these bodies in the performance of their tasks, the Minister of Education issues guidelines prepared by the State Schools Curriculum Committee .

Each state school has a *school board* (skolenaevn) which comprises three or five members; one member is chosen by the municipal council, the two or four others by the parents. The board supervises the school and organises co-operation between school and parents. It decides, upon recommendation from the teachers' council, what teaching aids and in particular what books are to be used by the school and it also determines the distribution of lessons among the teachers. If a parent or teacher wishes to challenge a decision made by the school board or school commission, they have the right to address either the municipal or, if necessary, county council; or ultimately address the Minister of Education directly.

Summarising influences on the recent development of school sex education, Danish informants regard the Ministry of Education commissions as having the strongest impact, with the following in descending order of importance:

local authorities, teachers' associations, parents' associations, other pressure groups such as the FPA, gay and feminist groups, and finally the media.

The Ministry of Education does heavily influence the content of sex education teaching, albeit in an advisory way. However, this is not as in Sweden where a central educational ministry commissions experts to produce standard manuals for use in all state schools (the vast majority). In Denmark, the educational materials, themselves, are created by individual authors and published commercially. It is for the head teacher of a school, a school board or a teachers' committee (or a combination of all) to decide on what is to be used.

Correspondingly, parents' groups have a right to decide on the materials employed in discussion with the school boards. This is a commune-level activity. It is likely to be the local educational authority which will decide upon the specific nature of the teaching in the schools of the commune. Nevertheless, teachers' associations and parents' associations (which, respectively, are ultimately representative of the whole of Denmark) are very powerful in influencing local and national government decisions - to the extent of having representation on all commissions. In recent years the opinions of representatives of sexual minority groups such as homosexuals have been taken seriously, though they have not actually sat on commissions.

It is remarkable that the system permits any form of central educational policy-making, standardisation of the curriculum, and standards-setting, though the high degree of social and political consensus in the country (compared with Britain) is an important factor in its success. Nevertheless, the democratic system might have been used to undermine the introduction of compulsory sex education in 1970. That this did not happen, in spite of sectional resistance was due to extensive government provision of a parallel private (fee-paying) school system alongside the 'Folkeskolen'.

There is no compulsory school education in Denmark, only compulsory education. Although few children are taught by their parents at home; around 10% of the school population are in private schools. Under the 1970 law, no sex education need be given in the private system. Moreover, the State supports private schools, subsidising them to 85% of their running costs.

As a result, parents who enrol their children at a private school do not in general have to bear heavy school fees. The Danish Parliament voted in May 1976 in favour of a proposal which would oblige municipalities to bear a large proportion of the cost of transport for children attending private schools. Primary education at private schools or at home must not fall below the standards laid down for State schools; it must cover the same compulsory subjects and be of comparable quality (supervised by the school commissions). The same applies to education given in the home.

Although some private schools are Christian-denominational, and do choose to opt out of state guidelines on sex education, most are merely 'elite' in the sense that they offer special facilities to pupils. They also conform, by choice, to the state guidelines on sex education. Nevertheless, it is this exceptional financial and other support for such an alternative system, which permitted the state to take the step of 'imposing' compulsory sex education on a democratic educational system. Although it has been well received (at least in principle) in the main, it nevertheless led to a unique event in which the Danish Government was force to defend its theory and practice of sex education before an international court of law (see below).

The Danish Sex Education Curriculum Guidelines

Before 1970, pupils in Danish schools were obliged to attend classes in the traditional subjects, special sex education being an optional subject demanding parental consent.

In 1960, the Curriculum Committee had published a 'Guide to Teaching in State Schools' which distinguished between instruction on the reproduction of man and sex education proper. The Committee recommended that the former be integrated in the biology syllabus while the latter should remain optional for children and teachers and be provided by medical staff. The Committee also advised guidelines for schools be drawn up on the contents of and the terminology to be used in sex education. This appeared in the form of a 1961 manual for teachers (*Sex Education in Primary and Secondary Schools in Denmark*) based on the Committee's report. This manual is different in style and substance than that which followed it in 1971. It is generally concerned with elaborating the underlying philosophy or rationale which justifies the recommended manner of dealing with issues of sexuality. Guidance is offered on the substance of what teachers are expected to provide to different age groups, with many, albeit implicit, references to preferred ethical positions, in the style of the Swedish *Instruction Concerning Interpersonal Relations*. The following gives the flavour of the guidelines of 1961:

> 'The pupils should be made to realise that in case of a premarital relationship, it must be an absolute condition that it means something serious, that you are true to the partner with whom you have chosen to cohabit, and prepared to accept your part of the burden should the association result in pregnancy'.(3)

The 1971 replacement for the 1961 guidelines : *Guidance on Sexual Orientation in the Danish Primary School* (produced by two of the three authors responsible for the 1961 version)(4), whose task was to provide guidance on the *compulsory* curriculum, shifts its emphasis correspondingly to 'methodological advice'. This appears in the form of rules for teachers which demarcate the rights and responsibilities of the teacher *vis-à-vis* the parent and medical personnel serving the school. The style is apologetic: '...it is not the intention of the school to take away anything from the home, but rather that the school would like to establish cooperation for the benefit of all parties'. (5)

It should be noted that this shift of emphasis was challenged by the authors contributing to the Curriculum Committee's work. The almost mandatory nature of this 'advice' ('teachers must not...)' suggests there was some apprehension, on the part of the state around this unprecedented venture of compulsory sex education in a society established on local autonomy. Neither the 1961 nor 1971 versions contain components of the knowledge base of the subject (as can be found in the Swedish handbook), this being left to the teacher to learn from other (commercial) publications. The philosophical and ethical objectives of the school programme take the following form:

'The objective of sex education shall be to impart to the pupils knowledge which could:

- help them avoid such insecurity and apprehension as would otherwise cause them problems;

- promote understanding of a connection between sex life, love life and general human relationships;

- enable the individual pupil independently to arrive at standpoints which harmonise best with his or her personality;

- stress the importance of responsibility and consideration in matters of sex.'(6)

Attention is paid to classroom technique, often in a high degree of detail (advisable length of lessons; use of slide projectors etc.). The following extracts provide a flavour of the 1971 guidelines, which commence with:

- description of the methodology of 'the concentric principle of instruction' (returning to the same field in successively greater detail as the child becomes older);

- the manner in which 'integration' of the subject can be managed;

- advice on 'conversational and debating forms of instruction':

'At all class levels, weight must be attached to trying to involve the class or group of pupils as a whole by using the conversational and debating form of instruction. On the other hand, the teacher should in no way convey sexual orientation to the single pupil which may assume the character of personal advice. On the whole the teacher must be advised *against* entering into a conversation or discussion of problems of a sexual nature with the single pupil outside the total group of pupils.'(7)

- terminological questions:

'Since instruction must be carried through on the general idea that the children should be spoken to in such a manner that their parents can feel secure about the form of the conversation, the teacher must be *advised against* using the vulgar terms in his instruction. It must be *recommended* that at the lower class levels he should use the conventional Danish designation.' (8)

- objectivity of ethical and social matters:

'The different points of view on sexual life confront the school with a rigid demand for objectivity in ethical and moral questions...it is assumed that the single teacher has a personal view which must be considered incompatible with the demand for objectivity in ethical and moral questions... the school must adopt a neutral attitude to the topics treated. The teacher must not identify himself with or dissociate himself from the conceptions dealt with. However, it does not prevent the teacher from showing his personal view (sic)... It must be possible for parents (from all social classes) to trust that the basic ethical points of view will be presented objectively and soberly.'(9)

- use of pictorial material (which must be restricted to line drawing rather than photographic);

- the limits of information about sexual behaviour, and the manner in which this is best approached:

'... it should be stressed that the teacher should not give information about the *technique* of sexual intercourse, nor should any other *technique* for the production of orgasm be treated in detail. As regards the form of instruction (it should be) based on purely objective conditions which can be described calmly, undramatically and completely seriously and with absolute respect for the pupil's self-esteem and self-confidence. Sentimentality, dramatisation of biological conditions, excessive gloominess or pathetic mention should be avoided since the pupils may feel it insulting and to some extent obtrusive. The topic should rather be treated with a touch of redeeming humour...' (10)

Recognising the position many teachers were placed in with the introduction of compulsory sex education, the guidelines also proposed that those teachers who feel they have insufficient knowledge should be able to attend special teacher training sessions. However, such measures were insufficient to prevent political events forcing changes in this bold educational step. By 1972, the Kingdom of Denmark had been challenged before the European Commission of Human Rights by families who contended that this measure violated both their Constitutional rights as Danish citizens, and contravened an Article of the European Convention to which Denmark was a signatory.

Partly because of these events, and doubts expressed by the National Association of Teachers about the workability of the regulations, in 1972 an amendment to the 1971 provisions revoked the compulsory element of teaching of sex education as a discrete subject in the 6th and 9th grades both for teachers and parents. More significantly, it further emphasised (see European Court ruling below) that teachers must convey this subject by strict reference to factual information and objectivity.

The Case of Kjeldsen, Busk Madsen and Pedersen versus the Kingdom of Denmark (11)

The applicants, three Danish couples with children of school age, lodged applications with the European Commission on Human Rights in 1971, against the Danish state. Following the 1970 Education Bill which, inter alia, had made sex education compulsory, these parents claimed that this violated Article 2 Protocol No 1 of the European Convention, defending their rights to hold the beliefs they had as Christian parents. For sex education invariably raised ethical issues which should be decided at home rather than school. However, they did not object to the teaching of sex education as such.

The case is worth reviewing in some depth here because it provided a unique legal forum in which the political-legal dilemmas raised by the subject, relevant to all European countries, were objectively aired. That is, the rights of the State *vis-à-vis* parents in the education of children for the common good. The resulting judgement provides a common philosophical and legal foundation for action by all states in the sphere of moral education.

The Case Against the Danish State:

The applicants claim that the alternative of private schooling is insufficient to fulfil the obligations of Article 2 Protocol No 1:

No person shall be denied the right to education. In the exercise of any functions which it assumes in relation to education and to teaching, the State shall respect the right of parents to ensure such education is in conformity with their own religious and philosophical convictions.

In particular:

- That this must be interpreted to mean that parents can exempt their children from sex education in public schools, because, unlike other subjects such as biology, it is impossible to offer value neutral sex education ('there is no such thing as objectivity in ethics').

- That there are insufficient private schools and that their pupils frequently have to travel long distances to attend them; and that the education therein may be inferior.

- That even the express wishes of the majority of parents cannot prevail against the terms of the 1970 Act.

- That minority religious views are as important as majority views; that 'many' people object to the liberal teaching of sex education at an early age in Denmark.

- That the guidelines which are intended to protect the interests of parents are merely optional, leading to a situation where many guidelines are ignored in practice by teachers.

The Response of the Danish State:

The reasons for the Government making the subject compulsory were:

- Because it felt that this was the only way to increase the effectiveness of the education as a defence of the population against the social welfare risks, and health costs of unplanned pregnancy, abortion and STDs.

- The logic of 'integration' within the school curriculum, in order not to violate the integrity of the subject by making it a specialism, meant that the entire school programme would be unworkable if parental right to withdraw the child was permitted.

- The teacher must follow a principle of 'ethical neutrality' when encouraging discussion of ethics:

  'The teacher should not identify himself with or disassociate himself from the views discussed. This does not however debar the teacher from voicing his personal opinion... Parents must be confident that the fundamental ethical views are presented in an objective and sober manner.' (1970 Act)

- Under the Danish Constitution, all parents have the right to free education in state schools, though they may wish to send their children to private schools, which are heavily subsidised by the state (or educate them at home).
- However, if the state school is chosen, the parents have a decisive voice in the administration of such schools. For example, they constitute a majority on the school board and if they object to a particular book or teaching aid it will not be used. The 'guidelines' issued by the Ministry of Education are only an 'assistance' to the school committees. The 'right' of education... by its very nature calls for regulation by the state, regulation which may vary in time and place according to the needs and resources of the community and of individuals.
- Specific sex education lessons which are recommended to be given in the 6th and 9th school years are voluntary, both for pupils and teachers.

The Outcome

The Commission, finding for the Danish State, concluded that the purpose of the Danish laws on sex education is not to impose on children a certain ethical or moral view of life. However, this conclusion was reached by a vote of seven against seven, with the President exercising his casting vote.

The Court case reaffirmed the 'factuality' rule: 'Danish sex education must by its nature rest on largely undisputed facts'(12) or the decision would have gone to the other side. However, the Court recognised the tenuous foundation on which the Danish case rested, and the apparent contradiction in that part of its defence which provided for alternative private schooling - an unnecessary provision if state school sex education could be, and was, everywhere truly 'objective' and 'factual'.

This point was taken up, in a separate opinion by Judge Verdross who in his dissent with the judgement drew a distinction between the communication of information on biology and natural sciences, on the one hand, and information concerning sexual practices on the other. The latter, he states, affects the development of the minor's conscience and, as such, may be violative of the parents' Christian convictions. Moreover, the Judge noted that the Danish legislation took cognizance of this distinction by providing private schools with the discretion to choose whether to include information on sexual matters although making biology courses, for example, mandatory. He stated that failure of the Danish Act to exempt children of parents with religious convictions at variance with these policies was, in his opinion, in derogation of Article 2 of Protocol No 1:

'...it seems to me necessary to distinguish between on the one hand factual information on human sexuality that comes within the broad scope of the natural sciences, above all biology, and on the other hand information concerning sexual practices, including contraception. This distinction is required, in my view, by the fact that the former is neutral from the standpoint of morality, whereas the latter, even if it is communicated to minors in an objective fashion, always affects the development of their consciences.'(13)

In spite of these flaws in the defence made by the Danish State, it is believed that the ruling of the European Court had a powerful and positive effect on Danish public attitude to the role played by schools in sex education. In particular, it alerted many parents to the need to exercise their rights in contributing to the school curriculum their children would be given. Initially, sections of the Danish media sided with the complainants over the principle of their rights *vis-à-vis* those of the state. However, media attitudes swung in the opposite direction when the case was coopted by minority religious interests in Denmark. In general, many parents did sympathise with the complainants. However, the case also launched a media analysis of the wider issues which eventually shifted public opinion to the side of the existing law. Although many were sympathetic to the rights of parents to educate their children without state interference, they were also realistic enough to appreciate the task that teachers fulfilled on their behalf.

Conclusions

The case against Denmark at the European Commission graphically displayed the difficulties confronting the state in a highly democratic society which finds it necessary for the common good to re-negotiate the historic rights of cultural institutions like the family. By however small a margin, it reaffirmed the right of the state to expose young people, through the state education system, to information with which their parents may not agree. The judgement nevertheless rested on the principle that it is valid for the state to take such measures in the face of exceptional social problems - in this case: STDs, unplanned pregnancies and abortions. The appearance of AIDS a decade after this court ruling adds weight to the position adopted by the Danish State.

It is to the credit of the Danish Ministry concerned that it confronted the issue of sex education realistically at the national level, by attempting to equip teachers with detailed guidelines, covering classroom methods by which they were compelled to infringe upon the historic role and rights of parents for the greater good. It would have been easier and even politically more expedient, simply to 'sub-contract' the whole task to local authorities, parents or teachers, or a combination of all, by decree, without concerning itself in the problems this shift of responsibility involves.

The central objective of the authors of the 1971-2 guidelines, currently in use, was to create a formula for compulsory education acceptable to the population. In redefining the boundaries of teacher and parent responsibilities, the authors created, firstly a detailed methodology for classroom practice, which revolved around the 'neutrality' principle; and secondly, defined the form the education should take: the 'factuality' principle. These steps have had some paradoxical consequences which the present National Commission is likely to consider.

Firstly, the 'neutrality' principle was *intended* to reassure parents that they would continue to have full jurisdiction over the moral guidance of their children in matters of sexuality. In theory, this principle is untenable - as some members of the European Commission took steps to point out (see the opinion of Verdross above). The provision of factual information about a subject permeated with moral issues charges this very information with a moral message.

Secondly, in practice, teachers' efforts to conform with the 'neutrality' principle has made Danish sex education the most liberal in the world *because* it is not perceived as the teacher's primary task to offer moral guidance in a particular direction; this being the job of the parent. As a result Danish sex education might be viewed by its European neighbours as excessively *amoral,* which is not what was intended.

It is also possible that guidelines based on these principles may have had the effect of demotivating as much as encouraging teachers. Because, contrary to the general principle of education in the case of this and all subjects they have been asked to avoid giving ethical direction. The same principle dominated Swedish sex education until 1977, at which time it was felt necessary to draw the distinction between fundamental and controversial values. Henceforth Swedish teachers would defend the former and operate according to the 'neutrality' principle regarding the latter. There is concern that the 'factuality' principle has deterred Danish teachers from dealing with the emotional element of teenage life. It remains to be seen whether a revision of the current guidelines will take the direction of Sweden, and what the public response will be.

Although not yet satisfied with the standard of sex education in Danish schools, educationalists feel that the introduction of compulsory education in the integrated style has nevertheless had a positive effect on the *level* of provision. One of the tasks facing the current Commission is to review the teacher training process and the quality of the sex education actually provided.

For it is still felt that too little is retained by pupils when it comes to protecting themselves for pregnancy at the right time. Other problems concern the difficulty of identifying sufficient time allocation to an 'integrated subject' (and the ease with which reluctant teachers can avoid confronting the subject properly within other subjects).

In common with its European neighbours, Denmark has still not adequately grappled with the problem of adequate teacher training (and therefore curriculum design in the college). Even having compulsory courses in sex education for student teachers is unproductive if they are insufficiently motivated to take the subject seriously or must follow a curriculum which gives priority to other subjects. Moreover, 'integration' (unless augmented by specific teaching) offers unenthusiastic teachers a mechanism to avoid providing such teaching at all.

Notes

1. Hoffmeyer ascribed to the philosophy behind the American study of child psychology by S Fraiberg: *The Magic Years* 1959.

2. see Braestrup, A *Sex Education in Denmark* Foreningen for Familieplanlaegning, Copenhagen 1973

3. Leth, I, Skalts, V and Hoffmeyer, E *Sex Education in Primary and Secondary Schools in Denmark* 1961 (English summary)

4. Hoffmeyer, E and Leth, I ibid.

5. English Translation: *Guidance on Sexual Orientation in the Danish Primary School.* The Curriculum Committee of the Danish 'Folkeskole' 1971 pg 16.1

6. ibid. pg 7

7. ibid. pg 10.1

8. ibid. pg 11.2

9. ibid. pg 14.1

10. ibid. pg 33.1

11. Council of Europe: European Commission of Human Rights *Case of Kjeldsen, Busk Madsen and Pedersen* Report of the Commission, Strasbourg 1975; Judgement 1976

12. ibid. Report of the Commission pg 46.

13. ibid. Judgement pg 27

Federal Republic of Germany: Creating Effective Structures of Consultation

Due to the federal political system of West Germany it is impossible to legislate nationally on such issues as education. The following describes the organisation of school sex education in the 'Land' or state of Hessen, with reference to relevant issues which have been decided federally in Bonn. What is outstanding in this country, and in Hessen in particular (as traditionally a liberal and progressive state), is the effort which has been exerted on devising local structures and methods to ensure maximum participation in the sex education curriculum design of the school (for example to define a division of labour between parent and teacher, and the mechanism by which they might constructively cooperate) while conforming to the principle that effective sex education based on the communication of accepted knowledge and social values should not be hindered by the idiosyncratic demands of individuals or movements.

Historical background

The evolution of (post war) state school sex education can best be understood, according to Plümer, by comparing three historical periods: the first saw the physical reconstruction of Germany following the collapse of the Third Reich. During this time, the FRG quickly emerged as a global economic power through the thrift and hard work of the partly refugee population. This period compares ideologically with 19th century Victorianism in its commitment to discipline, austerity and denial of pleasure. Internal cultural dissent was unknown. By the second period, during the 1960s, the FRG had become a highly industrialised state in which 'Victorian' values were rapidly becoming irrelevant. The ethic of consumption superseded that of production:

'It was in that relaxed moral climate of the so-called post industrial/capitalist society that the Frankfurt School of sociology identified the dynamics and consequences of the pleasure-based society, popularising a critical spirit around the meaning of many terms used without reflection (eg. health, freedom, education). Marx, Freud, Wilhelm Reich had a renaissance in universities and teacher training colleges. It was during this period that the so-called 'sexual revolution' took place.'(1)

The less glamourous side of the call for an end to sexual repression from the university and school students was the extensive commercialisation and 'commodification' of sexuality (sex-shops, sex cinema, sex-tourism, sex-articles).

In the third period, middle to end of 1970s, the subjects of ecology, pollution, (nuclear) energy and the threat of war became central ideological themes. It has been characterised by a widespread feeling of angst and helplessness. The catalogue of threats increased in 1985 with the arrival of AIDS in the public consciousness, reversing the previous period's emphasis on opening up human sexuality for exploration. What is known as 'Die Wende' - the political-ideological shift (from SPD domination to CDU/CSU) - heralded a re-affirmation of traditional moral values which took a form comparable to a similar shift in Britain: the ideological elevation of the family, and a reversal of 'progressive' attitudes towards abortion rights and sex education. This took a dramatic form in the FRG with the CDU/CSU administration destroying large amounts of educational literature ('Betrifft Sexualität') published by the SPD. Only in the 1980s is there perceived a 'thaw' in this reaction.

The Role of the German Family Planning Association

'Pro Familia' was formed in 1952 and spearheaded the establishment of family planning clinics across the FRG. It acquired a national status due to its role in campaigning for and helping to obtain a permissive abortion law, operating as a consumer organisation concerned with unplanned pregnancy and sexual counselling. Although a radical sex reform movement, it did not play a significant part in school sex education provision until 1970, as a result of the growing crisis of unwanted teen pregnancies.

In response, it instituted training courses for teachers, produced contraceptive information for young people, and advised *Land* governments who were establishing sex education regulations. This took the form of the presentation of *Pro Familia's* 'Theses on Sex Education' (1972 revised 1977): a series of progressive statements on theory and practice. In the late 1970s for practical as well as ideological reasons it withdrew from the school setting due to what it saw as an increasingly repressive political situation and a reduction in government funding for its work.

Principal Elements in Pro Familia's 'Theses on Sex Education' 1972/77

The theses offered a critique of traditional sex education principles: for example, that sex education must be oriented solely towards marriage/family, and must discourage pre-marital sexual intercourse:

'To delay, to divert and to repress a young person's sex drive is considered an essential contribution towards the development of his/her identity.'

The theses also questioned the (Freudian) premise that the development of culture is dependent upon repression of the sex drive:

'It is significant that most of the traditional books on sex education repress the second aspect of sexuality, the aspect of creating and receiving pleasure, by reducing sexuality to reproduction.'

The 'learning' (culture) theory of sexuality suggests sexuality can be formed and cultivated; a perspective which raises the need for sex education. *Pro Familia* recognises the psychoanalytic sense of the term 'sexuality' to refer to 'all libidinal wishes and contacts in all phases of human life', and rejects the sense of the term reduced to 'genitality'. The 'new' sex education denies the intrinsic merits of repression of sexuality (abstinence) and proposes that an important part of sex education is the critique of sex roles and the understanding of 'normal' and 'deviant'. It defends the right of the young to experience sexuality, though it challenges commercialisation of sexuality:

'Young people should be enabled to achieve satisfying interpersonal relationships (which include sexual ones).'

A second version of the theses, published in 1977, tones down their radical thrust, omitting the criticism of 'traditional' sex education, in particular its pro-marriage and family orientation. Nevertheless, the highly critical role prescribed for this school subject remained:

'Sex education acknowledges and examines critically how norms and customs are the result of historical and social conditions and thus might be changed'... 'Traditional conceptions of "typically female" and male behaviour must be changed, role stereotypes and the double moral standard must be attacked. Therefore alternative forms of living together must be recognised and supported.'

The theses were abandoned in 1984 as some sex educators found unsurprisingly that they brought them into too much conflict with schools and authorities in this more conservative period. *Pro Familia* withdrew from the field and now has no official stand on sex education. Ironically, the arrival of AIDS has created a new demand from schools for the services *Pro Familia* once offered, though the current political party coalition may remain unwilling to fund this libertarian organisation.

Political-Bureaucratic Structure

The Federal Republic is a union of states; cultural affairs are not decided at Federal level by central government, but subject to regulations of the *Länder*. In order to harmonise *Land* regulations on school affairs, the relevant ministers hold regular meetings in the form of the 'Kultusministerium Konferenze' (KMK): the Permanent Conference of Ministers of Education and Cultural Affairs.

With the balance of the two main coalition parties: Christian Democrats, Christian Social Union (CDU/CSU) and Social Democrats (SPD), neither gains an absolute majority. Since 1982 a conservative coalition of CDU/CSU-FDP (liberal) parties has been in power. The result is that few radical solutions can be posed, compromise being necessary. In sexual matters, a 'traditionalist' cautious path is taken, the government only taking initiatives if it is forced to by one of the composite parties or by public opinion (all changes of a sex reform nature having occurred during SPD rule). As sex education is not a matter for the Federal government, the only influence Bonn can exercise is through the Ministry of Youth, Families, Women and Health *(Bundesminsterium für Jugend, Familien, Frauen und Gesundheit)* by providing money for family planning and sex education publications, AIDS campaigns, and funding for the Family Planning Association, *Pro Familia*.

The one national body able to influence national provision of sex education is the 'Constitutional Court' *(Bundesverfassungsgericht, BVG)* - a supreme court able to overrule parliamentary and governmental decisions if they are believed to be out of step with the Constitution. The Constitutional Court ruled that all *Länder* provide general regulations which define the general learning objectives of state school sex education. Detailed guidelines could subsequently be created by the state Ministers of Education. Three *Länder* had created sex education regulations before the 1968 ruling (Hamburg, Berlin, Hessen); some have still to do so.

The Federal Role

The first legal regulations governing school sex education took the form of 'Recommendations on Sex Education in Schools' *(Empfehlungen zur Sexualerziehung in den Schulen)* in 1968, which were produced by the KMK. Considering the fact that this federal body has not only the option but is to some extent obliged to delegate responsibility for guidelines to the state level, it is remarkable that national governmental authority be given to regulations of such detail and balance. The essence of the ruling was that parents have a priority in this field of education, but that the school has a duty to supplement this role by the provision of 'objective' knowledge. In ruling that this education should permit the adoption of sex roles as men and women, and that heterosexual monogamy should be recognised as the cultural norm, the KMK were responding to a society feeling the impact of sexual reform, feminism and student unrest. However, it still managed to present a scientific and rational programme for schools which disregarded the extremes, as the following extracts reveal:

- Sex education is not to be taught as a special subject but integrated into biology, literature, social studies, religion.
- Sex education must be 'scientifically based'. The teaching of sex education must give a wide basis for discussion in the classroom.
- Parents must be informed about the *Land* regulations on sex education and the lessons planned by the teacher.
- Teacher training in sex education must be offered in the first phase of college curricula.

Similar to the Danish experiences, a federal court case brought by an individual family against a Hamburg school permitted a constructive revision and elaboration of federal regulations governing the relationship between the rights and obligations of parents *vis-à-vis* the school regarding this subject. Reviewing the case in 1977, the Constitutional Court identified the following guiding principles for all German schools:

- Individual sex education is in the first place part of the natural right of parents to educate their children (Article 6, Abs 2 GG). The state, however legitimately claims to carry out sex education in schools.
- Sex education in schools must be open to different value judgements and has to consider the parent's natural right, and their religious or ideological convictions. By all means, schools must refrain from any attempt to indoctrinate the young.
- In keeping with these basic guidelines, however, sex education is not dependent on the permission of the parents.
- Parents are, nevertheless, entitled to be informed well in advance of the contents and the methodical/didactic planning of how sex education is taught.
- By law, the legislator is obliged to decide upon the introduction of sex education in the school curriculum.

In sum, the sex education decided by the school has the same legal status as that given by parents. This constitutes an important defence against interference in what teachers decide is their teaching role and content in the agreement. The teacher is legally entitled to go beyond the limits of instruction (transmitting facts) into education (helping in the development of character, cognitive and emotive powers), having in view ethical aspects.

The BVG ruling is unique in Europe in specifically acknowledging the crisis which has developed around the knowledge base of school sex education (the limits of sexological scientific theorising versus normative education), in directing that a teacher cannot claim 'freedom of instruction and research' (Art 3 Abs 3 GG) as granted by the basic law to universities, or 'freedom of opinion' (Art 5 Abs 1 GG). These rights are restricted for him as a person teaching SE in a state school. On the other hand, parents cannot decide against sex education or to remove their children from the class.

Due to the Constitutional Court's decision, *Länder* school administrations have become more aware of conflicts, some establishing more elaborated guidelines to prevent them (eg. stressing the need of teachers to avoid what may be interpreted as indoctrination by parents, and to show discretion/tolerance towards religious/ideological convictions of parents).

The Hessen System

In Hessen a revised 'Law for the Administration of Schools' *(Schulverwaltungsgesetz SchVG)* was passed by the *Land* parliament in 1978. The passage on sex education reads:

> 'Sex education is undertaken as a teaching principle in various subjects. Through sex education, which as part of general education is one of the responsibilities of schools, pupils should be acquainted with questions of sexuality on a level suitable for their age. The aim of sex education is to enable young people to acquire an understanding of human and social partnership, especially within the marriage and the family, and to strengthen their feeling of responsibility. In sex education the appropriate discretion has to be kept as well as openness and tolerance have to be shown towards the various existing value-concepts in this area; any one-sided indoctrination is to be avoided. The parents have to be informed well in advance about aims, contents and teaching methods of sex education.'

In 1983, new 'Regulations for Sex Education' *(Rahmenplan und Richtlinien für Sexualerziehung an den allgemeinbildenden und beruflichen Schulen des Landes Hessen)* were decreed by the Minister of Education. These guidelines were based on the ruling of the Federal Constitutional Court, and in consultation with the spectrum of interest groups. The principle rationale behind this *Land* initiative is to create a system for teaching *which minimises the threat of conflict, lack of cooperation and trust between the interest groups*

141

concerned. This is seen to begin with consultation with parents by providing well in advance, information on the content of sex education. The structure of consultation in the state is of particular note, involving 15 members:

- one teacher (tutor in teacher training, biology) as chairman;
- one representative of the Catholic Church;
- three representatives of the Protestant Churches;
- two representatives of teachers' unions;
- one representative of the family planning association;
- one representative of the main personnel council of teachers;
- one representative of the main council of parents' representatives in Hessen;
- one representative of the Health Ministry (medical doctor);
- one representative of the Hessian Institute for Curriculum Planning (HIBS);
- one representative of the Hessian Institute for the Further Training of Teachers (HILF);
- one representative of the Hessian Council for Health Education (HAGE);
- one school psychologist.

This commission was established at the Hessian Institute for Curriculum Planning (HIBS). It did not receive Ministerial directions concerning the content of its task; the only condition being that its work must comply with: the 1977 decision of the BVG, and the 1978 Hessian law for the administration of schools.

The work of the commission was published in 1984. The following are extracts from this document (elements of which are relevant to the current British situation are in italics.):

Principles of Sex Education:

1. The Role of Sex Education within Total Education:

Sexuality provides people with many existential experiences: by loving a partner ...by taking on and fulfilling tasks and by promoting personal development; by gaining self confidence and by being confirmed by the partner; by bearing and educating children; by behavioural changes in the parents caused by a child, and by being a mother or father.

Sex education must include the biological, social and ethical areas of sexuality and take into account the emotional-affective as well as cognitive aspects.

2. The Objectives of Sex Education:

Sex education should influence in moral decision-making and behaviour in sexual relations. The objective should be -as with education as a whole- the free, sovereign individual who is aware of his/her responsibilities and has the judgement needed to make decisions in this area; but is also aware of his/her ties to and responsibility for the partner. *For this reason, sex education should also develop the understanding of the fundamental importance of human and social partnership, especially in marriage and then family,* and create and strengthen a sense of responsibility. Sex education should also make it clear to the young person that his/her full potential can only be attained by locating the sexual drive within social life. The intimate, personal sphere must be an area of freedom.

The same principles ...apply to sexual behaviour as to other areas of life: self-esteem, respect for the dignity and special characteristics of others, tolerance and mutual consideration *even if the sexuality of the other person is different from one's own.*

(Sex education has to take note of new scientific understanding of sexuality, which is changing attitudes and behaviour, particularly of young people; in so doing the religious and ideological principles of parents must not be violated.)

3. Areas of Sexuality:

The different subjects taught, teachers, parents and others to whom adolescents relate convey different aspects of sexuality. In order to achieve a united approach to sex education in school, different aspects have to be offered in accordance with teaching units of the subjects at hand. Therefore, coordinating conferences should try to determine key areas within each subject.

4. Cognitive and Emotional-Affective Aspect:

The psychological and sexual maturing of a child depends largely upon the mentality and behaviour of parents and educationalists... (tenderness or lack of it, interest or indifference, accessibility or inaccessibility, friendly or hostile approach to bodily matters)... The emotional aspect should (not) be ignored during school sex education: to convey only knowledge (=sexology) is asking too much of the student, especially if, at the same time, the objective is to enable him/her to make responsible decisions regarding sexuality. The teacher is further expected to teach: respect (the ability to let another person develop); responsibility (the ability/willingness to answer questions) distance (to avoid pressuring or attempting to control another); interest in the other person.

5. The Biological Area:

The biological questions in this area are taken care of in the specialist subjects during biology lessons through which students gain the factual knowledge required for a correct understanding of human sexuality (according to age, contraception and STDs have to be explained). Physical and emotional development are an inseparable unit. Thus, confinement to the mere biological approach to sex education is to be rejected. *The behaviour of the teacher, his/her understanding of the conflicts which may stem from the sex drive (desires, fantasies) during the psychosexual phase of puberty, is helpful to the student in order to find yardsticks for his/her own behaviour.*

6. The Social Area:

Sexuality is a largely non-specific basic human need, and among other things, is characterised by the fact that sensual feelings of desire can be separated from the biological function of procreation. *As human beings cannot rely upon their instincts and are subject to many influences, sexuality needs to be shaped and tied by norms and stabilised within cultural superstructures (regulations and institutions).*

Marriage is... an institution which serves to provide emotional security (endorsed by the Christian Churches as the basis for sexual fulfilment). The fact that many marriages end in failure... means that sex education in schools must help students to succeed in partnership and marriage. (The Hessen Constitution) demands that school sex education must aim to 'develop the understanding of human and social partnership especially within marriage and the family. Using historical and sociological perspectives on the changing relations of men and women,' a detached attitude should be developed towards wrong ideas of sexual performance and consumer temptation (the incorrect picture of sexuality drawn by the media).

7. The Religious-Ethical Area:

Sexual behaviour is to be judged by the same criteria as all other human behaviour: does it promote or hamper the ability of a person to give and receive love? In marriage and the family, one experiences the special 'I and You' relationship which realises in the best and most certain way the equality of men and women providing social welfare and legal security... despite the dangers of conflicts and misunderstandings. Within the range of school subjects, religious/ethical teaching has the special tasks of guiding the learning and maturing process from the child to adolescent.

8. Parental Rights and Educational Responsibility of the State:

Reference to the Hessen Constitution: 'The general responsibility of the school to educate children *does not rank below parental rights but is equal to them*... (to make an individual child into a responsible member of society)... Thus the state cannot be prevented from looking at sex education as an important part of general education... This applies in the first place merely to the teaching of facts and processes, which are conveyed in a value free way (ie. without relating to sexual ethics). But in principle actual sex education also falls within the schooling authority of the state... In general, schools have methods of teaching which are not available to the parental home... On the other hand education at home is more personal and direct. The school offers young people generally factual, scientifically-based information and comprehensive discussion... an additional help to complement the sex education in the home... education has to be given in "sensible cooperation".'

'the school cannot pretend to teach the children in all and everything.'

9. Sex education in classes with a high proportion of children from other cultural areas (especially Islamic):

'The teacher has to inform himself about the other cultural areas (eg. by taking special courses on sex education, through literature and by asking foreign colleagues and parents). During the teaching, itself, the different views on sexuality have to be treated with the required tact and tolerance in order to improve mutual understanding... The foreign children should be able to acquire the qualifications and behavioural patterns necessary for living in German society, and at the same time not lose the parental context of culture and tradition.'

Rules Governing the Implementation of Sex Education in Hessen

The teaching of sex education must be planned and implemented with the highest possible degree of agreement between parents and school. *The parents are entitled to be informed in good time about the content and methodological didactic form of sex education so that they are able to influence their children according to their own views and beliefs on the subjects which are being dealt with in the school.* Further topical subjects (eg. spontaneous questions by the students) can be dealt with by the teacher at any time. *Should a lesson follow (be constructed around a topical subject), the parents have to be consulted (in advance) via the advisory parents council of that class.*

In a conflict situation it makes sense initially to have a discussion between parents and teachers which can also be attended by the head and other specialist teachers.

It is believed to be important to create the ability for students to speak as a precondition for dialogue and learning, because of the lack of confidence about the appropriate language and taboo. On this matter the guidelines state:

'The use of inappropriate language ('street language') because of the inability to express oneself can be an obstacle to the creation of a partnerlike relationship and for the dialogue required for the solution of possibly existing sexual problems... If this obstacle is not removed by education , sex education in the meaning of these guidelines cannot be successful.'

'Planning and implementation of sex education for the individual age groups has to be determined at the beginning of the year by a *conference of teachers* involved. The class teacher or tutor is responsible for the implementation and coordination of sex education... or a teacher specially selected by the head. (However) Every teacher should be prepared to contribute to sex education according to the appropriateness of his subjects. If a teacher has justified (personal) objections this task can be delegated to another teacher after consultation with the teachers conference.'

'During the first two years at school, aspects of sex education in the parental home and school should be discussed at a *'parents' evening'*. In the following years, parents are to be informed in advance by the class-teacher or the coordinating teacher at parents' evenings about the intentions, content and media of sex education... Possible differences of opinion should be discussed by the participants with the intention of coming to an agreement.'

Participation and Exams: 'The students' reluctance to speak should be respected. There should be no oral or written exams in sex education because of the special emotive-affective aspects and values connected with the subject. This does not exclude finding out the cognitive level achieved by the student...requiring appropriate discretion...'

Interviews asking students intimate questions or any questions on their families are not permitted.

Teaching Media and Aids: 'Presentations in writing or in the form of pictures which are not orientated to the value system generally applicable in a pluralist society and outlined in the Basic Law are not suitable for use in teaching. This applies especially to products which hurt moral or religious feelings and have a degenerating and brutalising effect... it is not permissible to limit the sources of information in order to indoctrinate the student... *(Materials) can only be used in class after introducing them at a parents' evening and with the agreement of the parents concerned.*' (This has been extended to using parental donations specifically for the purchase of sex education materials - which become the property of those parents. Such a measure forestalls any attempt by individual parents to object to items used and builds confidence.)

Conclusions

The Constitutional Court's ruling on the separation of sexological discourse from sex education provides an essential criterion for the development of the sex education curriculum of schools. However, it remains for guidelines to be created to clarify the difference. Such guidelines have yet to be forthcoming, even though some Hessen schools have taken the initiative set by the *Land* guidelines to further develop conflict avoidance strategies of addressing controversial moral-sexual issues. These include: the formation of teacher sex education committees within the school on which a parents' council representative sits; and the development of more elaborated 'theses' on sex education for consideration at parents' meetings. There are also efforts to encourage the participation of senior pupils in deciding the content of lessons.

One highly effective conflict-avoidance strategy worthy of note is the use made of the German tradition of extra parental financial contributions to schools for the purchase of special educational or recreational materials. Such contributions have been used to buy all the sex education materials used in a school, which in effect become the property of the parents of each generation of pupils. This is expressed in the form of a stamp declaring that this is the case on each item ('property of the parents school council'). This simple device has allayed much anxiety and potential controversy about some of the more explicit education texts which must be employed in such education.

The Hessian guidelines are criticised because it is left to the teacher to decide what to take from contemporary sexology which does not 'violate the religious and ideological principles of parents'. Plümer makes the following observations on the efforts of this state:

> 'The representation of relevant groups in the commission, the compliance of the content with legal requirements, the checking of the draft paper by teachers, parents and ministerial departments, safeguarded from the beginning that the (guidelines) would be a 'middle of the road' paper...Its whole theme was conflict avoidance by various precise regulations... which seem to be useful steps for preventing or reducing conflicts.'(3)

The Hessian guidelines were developed in considerable detail by a highly representative commission of conservative and progressive authorities under the auspices of the *Land*. Although this work was undertaken in a relatively liberal period, these guidelines have survived, unlike much sex education orthodoxy in Britain, the shift in Germany to a more conservative Federal administration in the 1980s. This is as much a consequence of the structure devised to adjudicate on school practice as the content.

However, problems of practice remain here as in every other European country to date. For the state expects the teacher to conform with its designated requirements for the subject, however liberal, without sufficient teacher-training to negotiate the interests of: state, school, teacher, parent and pupil. Yet Plümer believes that models exist which may be used to resolve this problem with sufficient political will. This would take the form of an advisory service on which teachers could call to test out responses to situations arising in the classroom or in parents' meetings:

'There are some grave deficiencies in the organisation and training of teachers in sex education. In-service training courses can be effective but there are not enough of them. Sex education is not a school subject, it is a teaching principle integrated into various subjects. As sensible as the idea of integration seems to be, it is difficult to organise it in reality. Who is going to organise it? Even if sex education projects are organised for certain forms in a school, teachers are left alone without didactic -methodological assistance. Teachers have difficulty converting the global statements of the regulations into concrete curricula. There is obviously an urgent need for a comprehensive advice service, for a city or county, where teachers could turn for assistance (such advice services are established, for example, by the Churches for the teaching of religious education).' (4)

A recent survey of teacher opinion discovered that, although 11% of teachers interviewed said they thought their sex education qualification was sufficient, 66% considered it insufficient.(5)

There is a recognition, particularly as a result of the AIDS scare, that more systematic and further elaborated curriculum guidelines for sex education will be required. The Saarbrucken Ministry, for example, is currently replacing its 1971 CDU-created regulations with a set based on the Hessian model. Nevertheless, there are examples in Germany of a return to a conservative traditionalism, in the form of one state Minister (Gerhard Mayer-Vorfelder, Baden-Wurttemburg, Stuttgart) demanding that sex education again be confined to the transmission of biological facts.

In sum, in spite of signs of serious confrontation by the government(s) of some of the most difficult problems of school sex education theory and practice, many critics still feel there is much to be done. In a general review of sex education provision in the Federal Republic, Skaumal describes most guidelines as taking a path of 'problem avoidance' and preparation for marriage and family:

> 'there are hardly any reflections on learning objectives and contents... teaching is mainly conducted in a rational way with emotional avenues neglected'. Polls of students opinion which do exist suggest the emotional problems of human sexuality 'are utterly neglected'.(6)

Notes

1. Plümer, K-E 'Sex Education in Schools in the Federal Republic of Germany' in Meredith, P ed. *The Other Curriculum: European Strategies for School Sex Education* IPPF Europe, London, 1989

2. For example, in Sweden the teacher is expected to acquaint pupils with the latest scientific findings on sexology.

3. ibid. pg 19

4. ibid. pg 33

5. Gluck, G and Schliewert, H-J *Schule: der richtige Ort für die Sexualerziehung? Ergebnisse einer empirischen Untersuchung* RWTH Aachen, Sem. für Schulpsdagogik und Allgemeine Didaktik, Aachen 1987

6. Skaumal, U *Richlinien zur Sexualerziehung* IPN-Materialen, Kiel 1986

Chapter 6.4

Poland: The Survival of State Sex Education under the impact of National Politics

This and the country study following are included to display how the management of such an otherwise humble part of the school curriculum can echo differences and tensions in the wider society, around which political shifts occur.

Historical Background

For the first 10 post-war years, sex education did not exist either in the school or media, due to the traditional antipathy of orthodox Marxism to the subject of sexology. During a period of liberalisation between 1955-56, journalists attempted to bring to public attention many negative aspects of adolescent existence in the society of that time. It was argued that lack of provision for this age group by the State had led to a situation in which many young people sought escape from a society fraught by economic crisis through drug and alcohol abuse, and through sexual hedonism. Poland had evolved with a Marxist state philosophy superimposed upon a Catholic culture. This contradiction particularly in the area of family life has exacerbated the psychic and social alienation of Polish adolescents.

This alienation, combined with sexual ignorance, expressed itself among other ways, in high rates of unwanted pregnancy and abortion among adolescents. One response to this problem was the creation of Poland's Family Planning Association in 1957, with the original title, 'The Society for Conscious Motherhood' (SCM).(1) A group of physicians, journalists and teachers founded the society in Warsaw with the aims of informing about the harmfulness of abortion and the need for sex and contraceptive education.

In the early 1960s, the first sex education work of the society drew upon Swedish, German and even British theory and practice (in the latter case drawing upon the work of Cyril Bibby). The Family Planning Association thereby took on and retained a prime position in the development of school sex education in Poland. For example, on the initiative of the SCM, the 'voievodship' (province) of Lodz introduced a compulsory programme of school sex education in 1966, using a sex education programme created by M Kozakiewicz ('At the Roots of Sex Education'). This was followed by Katowice in 1970.

During the late 1960s and early 1970s, the FPA (whose name had changed to 'Family Planning Association', in Polish, TRR) was active in stimulating public and international debates on the theory and practice of the subject. Catholics and Marxists engaged in polemic, with the FPA proposing that there was little difference between the two in their puritanical attitudes to sexuality. Both Catholics and Marxists were resistant to the idea of sex education in schools, the negative attitude of the Soviet Union to issues of sexuality on ideological grounds inhibiting more open attitudes in Poland in this respect.

Nevertheless, during this time, the first sociological researches on the sexual behaviour of Polish adolescents were conducted, and clinical sexology was established as an academic discipline.

Until 1970, the TRR's undertakings, and in particular those of its sex education committee, enjoyed the favourable but rather passive support of school authorities (it was strategically useful for the authorities to have a separate non-governmental organisation specialising in this subject than to involve themselves in this subject and produce confrontation with the mighty Catholic Church). However, in 1972, the Ministry of Education sponsored a TRR-designed curriculum guide for teachers, the contents of which drew upon otherwise unavailable foreign material. Before this time, teacher training courses had no sex education component of any kind.

'1970 was not only the time of dramatic change of the ruling team but also a very radical change in the attitude of the ruling centre to the family, education of youth, and consequently to preparation for marriage and family life. The turning point was the year 1973, when the Party adopted a special resolution on the topic (Giereck coming to power)... They have created a special discrete subject: "Preparation for Life in the Socialist Family", wishing to show that a truly new era is beginning in the education field with the coming of the Giereck administration.'(2)

The economic crisis in the mid-1970s led to a political manoeuvre in which the State sought the support of the Catholic Church. This led to tactical support for the Church's anti-family planning, pro-natalist position, leaving the FPA without official support. A course entitled 'Preparation for Family Life', introduced by the FPA in 1974 as an optional subject for more than 2000 schools, was increasingly challenged and modified through pressure from the Church, which argued its contents were contrary to Catholic conscience and teaching. At its lowest point, the FPA was virtually bankrupted through the efforts of the Church-State alliance - a development assisted by the 'Solidarity' movement. By 1981, the FPA's 'Preparation for Family Life' course for schools had been banned completely.

In the early 1980s, a shift in the political climate through the efforts, among other social scientists, of economists pointing to the depressive effect on the economy of a rising population, led to increased government sympathy for sex education. By 1984, so rapidly had opinion turned in the FPAs favour that a new Ministry of Education decided to make 'family life education' (of an FPA variety) compulsory in all schools, beginning in 1986. Ironically, the enthusiasm of the new Minister of Education for an FLE programme has led to the production of a liberal sex education text for adolescents which has scandalised adult opinion in Poland. The more cautious FPA is seeking to have revisions made in this publication to increase its 'respectability' and acceptability among the Catholic public. It has also produced, during 1987, its own manual for teaching practice aimed at the professional.

The Development of the Sex Education Curriculum for Schools

The programme for primary schools (age 7-14) in 1959 contained information on plants and animals without reference to human reproduction. By 1963, human reproduction began to appear in the general curriculum. During the period up to the 1970s, a narrow version of sex education advocated by medical doctors prevailed, which approached the subject as a pedagogical exercise: transmission of facts in appropriate ways to equip pupils with a stock of knowledge on the physiological, psychological and sociological side of sexual, marital and family life. The implicit methodology was descriptive.

The 1970s saw an expansion of the influence of the FPA and a clarification of the concept of sex education in a more normative direction: preparing young people for understanding the problems they would encounter in their sexual lives:

'We are in favour of a wider conception of sex education, although it is much more difficult to realise. Such education should be used to shape the personality of the pupil in regard to his attitude towards others and in his adoption of marital and family roles.'

This statement contains the proposal that although such education will be limited by the conditions imposed by the context of the classroom, it must aim to address matters of family life which have little directly to do with sexuality as such. The way these matters must be addressed must conform with society's expectations of the next generation.

This pursuit of the ideological 'middle ground' by the FPA, although couched within contraceptive rights for adolescents, was not reflected in the events of the 1980s, when supporters of the Catholic Church sought to eliminate the pedagogy of the FPA. Recalling this time, Krzysztof Kruszewski (Professor of Pedagogics; former Minister of Education 1980-81) has noted:

152

'At the outset of the turmoil, the "Teachers' Solidarity" (movement) focussed its efforts on social and political demands connected with wage claims... later this included pedagogical claims and demands. One of them was the elimination of "ideologically based subjects" (including) family life education. "Solidarity", with great haste, proposed an alternative curriculum, "Preparation for Life", based on almost 100 percent Roman Catholic views and literature. This programme was negotiated with the Minister, who felt himself obliged under the political pressure of this movement to suspend the (existing) family life education lessons.'(3)

The return of sympathy for the FPA approach during the mid-1980s has led it to seek ways of reconciling its position with the Catholic opposition. One way in which this has been achieved has been through a cooperation on a publication for teachers' use which sets out the FPA and Church approaches to controversial ethical issues side by side for the reader to judge. Members of the Catholic Church have cooperated in this venture in spite of objections from Church officials because of a recognition of the need for dialogue on that side.

The FPA approach to sex education with its emphasis on family life has brought the support of Polish trade unions. The cause of sex education has also been fought by Polish sexologists, who have had an enormous impact on the medical profession.

Details of the Curriculum for Secondary Schools

Since 1986, the government has decreed that schools must provide at least 2 hours per month of sex/family life education. The following is an excerpt dealing only with issues of sexual, marital and family life, taken from this programme:

Course 1 Grades i and ii (age 15-16 years):

Part 1: Erotic Life:
- psychosexual development as a component of individual development;
- the conditioning and development of the sex drive;
- love and emotions and their social-historical conditioning;
- juvenile erotic relations and their moral status;
- psychosexual maturation (differences between the sexes) in adolescence;
- models and ideals of love; cultural definition of attractiveness;

- sexual activity in juvenile relations; responsibility;
- physiology of reproduction and methods of contraception;
- physiological and moral/social consequences of abortion.

Part 2: The Family:
- juvenile ideals of marriage and family;
- family law and codes;
- counselling assistance;
- motherhood and fatherhood; pregnancy and childbirth.

The Government's Sex/Family Life Education Programme (taken from the manual, 'Wychanowie' 1987)

1. Sex education and family life education issues and topics:
- implementation of family life education;
- cooperation with parents, organisations and institutions (to facilitate the implementation of the subject);
- the aims and goals of FLE;
- psychosexual and emotional development of the individual;
- social conditioning of sexual behaviour;
- different types of sex education.

2. Practical examples of communicating the more difficult topics to students:
- methodology for the handling of typical sexual questions and problems posed by pupils;
- methodology for dealing with non-typical problems of young people in specific life-situations;
- the first days of marriage;
- the art of marital cohabitation;
- sexual cohabitation in marriage;
- how to communicate in marriage;
- on fidelity and jealousy;
- understanding, managing and solving marital conflicts;
- family planning.

Conclusions

The evolution of sex education in Poland has not differed substantially from other Western European countries, insofar as its progress has been exceptionally rapid in the post-war years, beginning with the ideas of a few medical professionals and educationalists. During the last 30 years, such education has developed according to the cooperation the FPA could maintain with the national Ministries of Education and Health. However, implementation in the classroom has been dictated by the willingness of head teachers to absorb this subject into the school curriculum.

Until recently, with the exception of periods in which the Church became dominant, guidelines for school practice have been created almost exclusively by the FPA, 'sub-contracted' to undertake this task by the government Ministry. However, the recent zeal of government to pursue this subject more enthusiastically has appeared in the form of a law making the subject compulsory for all schools, and the appearance of a government publication created and circulated publicly without the editorial advice of the FPA (though with some contributions from FPA member experts).

In few other countries can the evolution of school sex education have been so directly and inextricably connected with national politico-cultural events in this country's recent history - particularly due to the centrality given to national morality and demography (poor work effort in the national economy put down to poor family relations). This has taken the form of shifting governmental enthusiasm, then periodical resistance to form the subject is given in the school curriculum, depending upon the wider moral-political interests it has had to negotiate to maintain power and legitimacy. It is difficult not to compare this with recent events in the UK. What is perhaps special to Poland, due to economic extremes, is the fact that successive Ministries of Education have sought to endorse enthusiastically programmes of sex/family life education in pursuit of a national reputation for 'progressivism' over the previous regime .

Notes

1. see Kozakiewicz, M, 'The History and Politics of Planned Parenthood Laws in Poland' in Meredith, P & Thomas, L eds *Planned Parenthood in Europe* Croom Helm, London 1986 pg 197ff.

2. Kozakiewicz, M 'Sex and Family Life Education through the Polish School System' in Meredith, P ed. *The Other Curriculum: European Strategies for School Sex Education* IPPF Europe, London, 1989

3. ibid.

Chapter 6.5

Belgium

The European examples described in this study have been included primarily to identify methods used in other countries to overcome common obstacles to sex education practice in schools. A brief description of the situation pertaining to Belgium displays how its political history and culture has created impediments to the standardisation of school provision of controversial aspects of the curriculum which far outweigh those created by political parties in Britain.

Historical Background

Revisions of the Belgian Constitution between 1970 and 1980 have replaced a unified legislature and government with a highly complex system of powers given to the cultural and linguistic communities (French-, Dutch-, and German-speaking). While the major division within Belgian society might be regarded as linguistic, an equally important division stems from Catholic versus non-Catholic, including secular persuasion.

The division of the Belgian school situation into two major blocs is deeply rooted in Belgian political and cultural history, feelings about which remain so intense that it is unlikely Belgium will ever see any standardised sex education curriculum agreed for the whole country. This is likely to impede efforts to improve the quality of provision in the community as a whole. Seeking control over the school system has been a major preoccupation of Roman Catholics and humanist free-thinkers since the last century. 'Freedom' of education was and remains the principle behind the organisation of education along two lines.

The first *Primary School Act* 1842 and *Secondary School Act* 1850 made Roman Catholicism compulsory in all schools irrespective of the affiliation of the pupil's family. By 1878 a radical Liberal Party came to power with the objective of bringing the school system under the control of the State in order to limit the power of the Roman Catholic church. Efforts to make the RC religion optional produced a Catholic backlash orchestrated from Rome, to which the administration responded by breaking off diplomatic relations with the Holy See (1880). Following demonstrations and social disruption, the RC religion was reimposed in 1895. By the end of the 19th century, this conflict was settled periodically by the Catholics and Liberals declaring their own interpretation of the Belgian Constitution. However, the battle over control of the school system re-emerged after World War II, as efforts were made to permit the population the option of Catholic or secular education in the form of reducing grants to the Catholic system.

Following changes of government during the 1950s, a National School Commission was created as a compromise between the 3 main political parties. A resulting 'school pact', inter alia, permitted State schools to offer a choice between a religious ethics course and one of 'non-confessional ethics'. As Deven describes, teachers must henceforth conform to a 'neutrality' principle not merely restricted to issues of sexual morality:

'Teachers in State schools can take no sides about social or ideological issues which divide public opinion. They cannot show favour to any particular religious or ethical system. Exception is obviously made for teachers of "religion" or "ethics", although they too have to shun critique of others' tenets or dogmas.' (1)

Making a peace by means of a 'school pact' has been achieved at great financial cost and through a guarantee of non-interference in the separate school systems, and in the provision of funds for parts of the country to create education facilities which equally serve the different parties.

There is a Minister for Education for the two linguistic communities. Any matter labelled 'ideological' (viz: sex education) is delegated to the autonomous decision-making of school governors. Predictably, the Belgian Parliament has never debated sex education, it being mentioned only as a panacea for other issues of national concern such as contraception or abortion.

Where there have been broad initiatives which hinge upon the theory and practice of sex education (eg. coming from the universities or mass media), the mechanism of advisory boards within the separate school systems become immediately involved, having the effect of delaying, dismissing or diluting anything which appears to run against their own specific ideological interests.

The management of sex education in schools can only be clearly discussed in connection with the Catholic school system compared with the State school system, even though other smaller systems coexist (schools governed by municipalities and provinces).

Initiatives of the State and Catholic School Systems (Dutch-speaking community)

State schools have been concerned to assist teachers in terms of guidance as well as protection since the 1950s. This took the form of a manual for teachers of 'ethics' authored by the Chief Inspector of moral education and two teachers. In 1973, a Minister of National Education (W Calewaert) created a commission (which contained teachers and FPA members) to provide guidelines on sex education. The resulting report recommended a scientifically-based integrated sex education. A consequent discussion of the findings resulted in a plea for the development of an integrated and emancipatory school subject designed with the participation of all relevant interests. This initiative failed as a result of change in government, though a commission for sexual and affective guidance continues to function as a result of Calewaert's endeavour. During the 1970s, it was responsible for the creation of audio-visual materials which are used in some Catholic as well as State schools. The Minister for Education serving the subsequent 1981 Christian Democrat-Liberal administration has not maintained and even discouraged this initiative. The country's lack of political continuity with successive replacements of Ministers of Education with their own programmes has militated against continuity of policy measures of the above kind.

Within the Catholic system, until recently the clergy have dominated the school governing bodies, under the general direction of a National Secretariat. Through its pedagogical bureau, it creates guidelines and recommendations which are delivered through a 'General Council for Catholic Education' (ARKO), though individual Bishops intercede on issues within their own diocese. It appears that the Catholic school administration has pursued guidelines on sex education with some vigour. In 1967, a 'Catechetical Commission for Secondary Schools' was created by the Belgian episcopy, which, over 3 years created a curriculum according to age and educational level. Reflecting the spirit of the Second Vatican Council, the commission noted the need for a responsible sex education to suit a changing society. Cooperation with parents and teachers of biology is recommended. Over the 1970s and 1980s, these curricula have been endorsed by the Bishops and teachers' representatives and have become available for use in schools. They conform essentially to the teachings of the Church, particularly with respect to contraceptives.

This was reflected in the reaction of the Director-General of the National Secretariat for Catholic Education to the 1987 information campaign on AIDS created by the Secretary of State for Public Health. A letter was circulated to all school governors and head teachers labelling this campaign as too permissive. Deven perceives the AIDS issue as highlighting the increasing difficulty facing the Catholic school system from operating a strategy of educational isolation from other influences in Belgian society. Such pressures are likely to lead to the operation of 'hidden curricula' of a more liberal or realistic type, depending upon the governors or head teachers of individual schools. In such a context, more elaborated guidelines for practice would only impose a more rigid sex education.

Events Relating to Sex Education in the Francophone Community

In 1970, in reaction to the progressive (youth) culture of that period, the Socialist administration of Abel Dubois, established a 'mission' or special committee, comprising teachers of various disciplines, to identify an educational formula to address the sexual and emotional needs of young people in secondary and higher education. The resulting programme was conceived of as transcending the normal definition of education to refer to nurturing of autonomy and responsibility in this age group. In 1977, a Catholic Minister for National Education (Louis Michel) proposed to dissolve this committee, prompting a reaction from political figures and organisations such as the Francophone branch of the Belgian FPA. As a result of media attention, the measure was delayed until 1978. Nevertheless, it is believed that the activities of this 'mission', in addressing problems of sex education, had an effect on the general philosophy of education of State school programmes in general. This is perceived in a 'manifesto' published by the Francophone Ministry of National Education in 1986, which reads:

> 'The educational programmes which the Education Communities are requested to establish are demanding. They must be aimed at making the school an instrument:

- to transmit structured and coherent knowlege;
- to develop attitudes which are in line with the values adhered to by the community;
- to develop the personality of each pupil, taking his aptitudes and interests into account, as well as the needs of the community;
- to awaken in each pupil an awareness of the responsibility he has to develop in his own life;
- to provide equal opportunities for all by taking differences between pupils into account.

> In accord with a liberal interpretation of education, the authors of the "mission" had proposed that:

- It has been decided to consider sexual and emotional education as part of general education.

- Priority should be given to emotional, ethical, and social problems. Scientific knowledge should be drawn upon in order to explain sexual and emotional behaviour.

- Young people should be encouraged to air and understand problems experienced in the sexual and emotional life. We are confident that the confrontation of different ideas and opinions on the basis of a profound knowledge of the values underlying them can enrich the study of a human problem, improve ethical judgements, and make the options of emotional life clearer and more responsible...

- To give some examples, the values of the couple, the family, and procreation are affirmed, to be sure, but this does not rule out the study of behaviour and problems relating to: celibacy, premarital sexual relations, choice of contraceptives, divorce problems etc.'(3)

This report also mentioned the need for teacher training to cover the above and the role which could be played by the FPA in this regard. In 1978, a Ministry of National Education press conference announced that: the psycho-medical-social counselling (PMS) centres 'will henceforth assist teachers and parents in their educative task'; that these changes will be defined in law; and that the PMS centres would take on the sex education role which had been previously left to visiting lecturers.

These deliberations had the implication that a greater number of people would be involved in assisting all schools to provide for sexual and emotional education. However the pronouncements would come to nothing, due to the fact that the political structure affecting school sex education remained unchanged. Power remained centred in the school boards, ever unwilling to displease parents, and who were free to refuse such assistance.

Aronis-Brykman contends that in spite of the above, the family planning centres have been permitted to give increasing numbers of lectures in (State) schools during the 1980s, albeit in 'moral science' classes. (4) There is little information available concerning which is provided under the title, 'sex education' in the Catholic school system.

Conclusions

For the operation of the complex Belgian political administration of schools to be possible, it is necessary to 'sub-contract' the curriculum design of ideological subjects to what Deven calls 'private initiatives', that is those movements whose *raison d'être* is the promotion of a stance independent of the ideological stance of one or other communities.

Each organisational power (the RC Church and the State) autonomously dictate the conception of the subject at the school level. In practice this means that it is forced either into 'religious teaching', a branch of RC ethics (Godsdienst), or non religiously aligned ethics (Zeedenleer) in the State system *by nature of the political organisation of education in (Dutch-speaking) Belgium*; a compartmentalisation which does not acknowledge, even in theory, the integrity of the subject in its own right. More likely is sex education to remain located in a primarily medical-biological paradigm as a solution to these political complications.

A survey conducted by the pharmaceuticals manufacturer, Organon in 1987 revealed that teachers were concerned with self-censorship in relation to this subject, feeling uncertain about the reactions of school governors, parents' committees and their head teachers. Moreover, in the spirit of a self-fulfilling prophesy, teachers, in general, are not believed to be the most appropriate persons to provide sex education, due to their poor motivation, lack of the special interpersonal skills for this subject, and fear of the reaction of superiors. Predictably, pupils, when surveyed, also perceived their teachers as ineffective in this field.

Exceptional regulations, for example those relating to the arrival of AIDS, are created and integrated into 'sex education' separately, according to the programmes of the two school systems. Nevertheless, where national commissions have come close to addressing ethical problems connected with education, they have been unable to address the issues directly (ie. create an appropriate agenda).

Keeping in mind that the Belgian FPA is a 'federation' of organisations representing the two linguistic communities, there have been attempts by its members to provide lectures in schools at the request of individual head teachers, and to create training courses for teachers, irrespective of affiliation. The FPA branches concede that it is more realistic to pursue initiatives in sex education which do not depend upon the school setting: for example through the TV medium or through the activities of youth organisations.

Notes

1. Aronis-Brykman, H and Deven, F 'Sexual and Affective Education in the Belgian School System' in Meredith, P ed. *The Other Curriculum: European Strategies for School Sex Education* IPPF Europe, London, 1989

2. ibid.

3. ibid.

4. ibid.

Chapter 7

Prerequisites for School Sex Education in a National Curriculum

This study has attempted to chart the process by which the state has become involved in the moral education of young people in matters of sexuality and relationships. Using the method of 'de-construction' sucessfully directed at other social phenomena (for example the critique of sociobiology), this study extends a bridge to wider and more sophisticated frameworks for the analysis of cultural change. Here the route has been taken of comparing historical developments in Britain with a number of European countries which have confronted, with more and less success, problems similar to those in this country. In spite of differences in culture and politico-economic systems, there are remarkable similarities in national efforts to establish systems for the teaching of sex education through schools, and the kind of impediments which must be surmounted. There are important lessons in these experiences for Britain.

What has been revealed is the intensely (national) *political* character which the management of school sex education takes on, in spite of the ethical, philosophical and administrative issues which dominate the classroom context. This being so, it has been argued that problems of practice can be resolved satisfactorily only through corresponding national political measures, which can neither be delegated or 'sub-contracted' easily in the system dealing with health/education affairs for schools. This goes some way to explaining the difficult role which was taken on by the (necessarily non-political) family planning association since the war.

The evolution of school sex education in Europe displays various forms of governmental manipulation often as a means of mediating between competing interests, though also in defence of its own interests of a wider political, demographic and even economic kind. Unfortunately this manipulation is seen to impede the development of standards for the subject as much as facilitate them. What is clear is that progress in school curriculum development can not be achieved without the mandate given to the government.

Although this country has so far escaped the kind of religious-secular antagonisms which must be endured by some governments (eg. Belgium or Poland) which have attempted to promote an ethics suited to pluralist, modern, urban industrial societies, Britain seems to have been especially burdened by the often irrational politics of the party in its pursuit of the most rational and workable system of nationally-standardised (moral) education in sexuality and relationships. In one period during the last 20 years, the pragmatic philosophy of 'causalism' seemed to provide a workable means on which to create legislation on matters of sexual morality which did not stimulate destructive ideological confrontations between the opposing political lobbies. Davies has referred to 'causalism' as the only possible language of communication between the ideological forces found in Parliament - the proposition that laws (or systems of education) might be organised at least to minimise the harm or suffering some citizens would undergo within the existing moral status quo.(1) In terms of political mobilisation, this meant gaining the support of the 'middle ground' for social policy measures of a traditionally controversial nature. Unfortunately, as far as the development of sex education is concerned this foundation was short-lived; the subject has all but returned to being the property of the party.

The administrative measures recently introduced by the Conservative party to re-locate responsibility for sex education in the school curriculum to the school governing body represent, at face value, an attempt to democratise the decision-making process, particularly in the direction of parents. Unfortunately, for its own political reasons, this measure was explicitly designed to marginalise the teacher - the very professional whose task it is to 'deliver' the subject at hand. However politically expedient *vis-à-vis* interest groups, which must be served, it has merely exacerbated the problem of discovering a means to secure the commitment and enthusiasm of school teachers.

On the other hand, more auspicious for the *future* of this subject has been the government's creation of a national curriculum, which establishes the principle of *national standardisation* of the contents of school education. In a more appropriate political climate, the logic of this development will be to extend the national curriculum to include non-core subjects including health/sex education. The very controversial nature of this subject makes this necessary, as events in other European countries reveal.

What is common to European experiences of including sex education in the state educational systems?

Firstly, there exists, irrespective of political system, *a universal tension of 'traditionalistic' versus 'progressive' tendencies*, which appear around matters of moral socialisation of the young outside the home. This tension has individual psychological roots connected with the conscious articulation of sexuality, as well as rational 'political' causes. It has been increased as a result of recent developments in the science of sexology in which the traditional 'factual' basis of sexual behaviour has undergone 'de-' and 're-construction'.

Thus, Foucault has argued that, 'What we lack is not a... truth but a way of coping with a multiplicity of truths' (sexual pluralism). It has to be recognised that sex 'education', even the provision of information, can have subversive implications for traditionally fixed sexual categories, interpretations, roles and identities. These include: 'adolescent feelings', prejudice, joy, desire, the erotic; masculinity, femininity; racism/sexism, homosexuality, power/authority, domination/submission. The emergence of critical sexologies, and the political reaction they create, makes it imperative to clarify the differences between sexology and school sex education - with reference to their respective functions, purposes and limitations.

The school can undertake a small part of what 'sex education' includes, though in the absence of any national curriculum planning in this field, schools continue to provide, on a trial and error basis, a subject without boundaries but permeated with risks. European experiences offer examples of classroom strategies which offer the teacher a refuge from allegations of value-bias while communicating basic values incorporated into all school education.

Britain has yet to establish a national authority with the means and legitimacy to deliberate on the theory and practice of sex education *vis-à-vis* sexology, as has begun to occur in other European countries. The terse and guarded 'guidelines' offered to local education authorities and schools through the occasional pamphlets of the Department of Education and Science (2) do not compare with the serious and systematic efforts undertaken there.

Secondly, those European countries in which most progress has been made in removing controversy from the subject have all found it necessary to draw upon the moral and regulatory authority of *national government* (at least in the form of a national commission divorced from party politics), in conjunction with local participation in the design and implementation of school programmes. This involves identifying a 'correct' role for the respective levels of authority from Ministry to classroom. A *sine qua non* of this process is the identification of specific interests common to the Ministries of Health and Education - bodies which display ideological antagonism in all countries reviewed. It is the antithesis of 'sub-contracting' as a convenient political strategy for authorities to avoid becoming involved in matters of potential controversy which may constitute threats to their wider interests.

To date, British governments have resisted pleas to address the problems of sex education theory and practice with a view to absorption into a core national curriculum.(3) It has been politically far safer to 'permit' individual education authorities and schools to make their own arrangements. Yet, as Doggett has noted:

> 'Without guidance from above, few education authorities or individual heads have regarded sex education as a priority area, and many schools have "officially" ignored the subject, while "unofficially" allowing those staff who feel comfortable and concerned enough to approach it as they see fit'...'The virtual autonomy of LEAs in curricular matters has resulted in much diversity of practice and content.' (4)

Thirdly, representative commissions of inquiry, whose task it has been to address the major issues of theory and practice, create the *agenda* by which sex education can be understood and communicated. Identifying the agenda fulfils two important functions: it provides a basis for communication of the major issues of controversy to a range of audiences, providing a 'language' and body of information. It should also provide educators with the means to create guidelines for the negotiation of the more sensitive and difficult aspects of the curriculum *vis-à-vis* other interested parties (such as parents, the Churches, the media). In addressing the items of this agenda, the commission would be forming the basis for a national standard of teacher training as well as creating guidelines for classroom practice established with the inputs of a wide range of interests.(5)

Creating an Agenda for a National Commission: in Britain, such an agenda has yet to be established. It would be with reference to such an agenda that a National Commission would seek to establish guidelines for sex education, would be complete without reference to issues of content and methods of the teaching of this subject which have been sources of recurrent anxiety and controversy in Parliament (see chapter 2). The following points summarise the principal areas of concern:

Issues of content:

1. The relationship between fundamental and controversial values, and the distinction between such values: the 'factual' component of teaching, and the place of personal opinion and the avoidance of 'indoctrination'. This would include the respective rights and responsibilities of: the school system, parents, the state, and the pupil around key issues (eg. fidelity, pre-marital sexuality, forms of cohabitation, contraception etc). See Sweden's distinction between the handling of 'fundamental' and 'controversial' values versus Denmark's defence of the 'neutrality' principle.

2. A weighing of the evidence (statistical and social-ethical) relating to the health cost/benefit ratio of sexual activity and contraceptive practice in adolescence, in relation to unplanned pregnancy.

3. Guidelines on teaching on the subject of homosexuality and the rights of sexual minorities. This would cover the subject of sexual deviation, pornography etc. The distinction between information about and advocacy of sexual lifestyles.

4. Approaches to discussing sex roles, marriage and family life, sexual discrimination (including the management of multi-ethnic/cultural audiences (see Sweden).

5. The political implications of scientific sexology and 'sex reform'. Identifying level of education in sexuality and personal relations relevant to different ages and audiences.

Issues of teaching method:

1. Establishing criteria for designing/assessing teacher training and performance. The creation and allocation of necessary financial and material resources.

2. Establishing, at the school governing body-classroom level, a structure for consultation and decision-making authority in deciding curriculum content and design.

3. The issue of all or part of sex education being optional/compulsory for teacher and pupils. (Mandates are worthless and even counter-productive if they produce only nominal compliance with guidelines, however good.)

4. The rights of parents regarding choice of content and pupil attendance.

5. Guidelines for classroom practice methods: rules for the protection of teacher and pupils; privacy and self-disclosure.

There have been some attempts to create guidelines which cover some of the above items. However, they have come primarily from interest groups on the right which do not, and cannot hope, to represent anything more than a small section of British society.(6) In 1972, Dallas found that in British sex education to date, the integration of the subject across the curriculum has led to duplication and inconsistency, and from the inability of schools to integrate their physical and emotional approaches to the subject.(7) Doggett contends that little has changed in this regard:

'With such a plethora of courses and subject areas which could include sex education, it would seem obvious that coordination is essential if wasteful duplications and/ or damaging ommissions are to be avoided. Yet in 1984, Dixon observed that "few schools appear to have any policy discussions on sex education and teachers are unsure". ...Dallas felt that there was a strong case for a coordinator to spend much time "just becoming familiar with the mass of material" and producing a synthesis best suited to the school.'(8)

The National Council of Women of Great Britain have also argued that sex education should have a core curriculum component to avoid problems of duplication and omission.(9) How could such a task be undertaken?

There are a variety of administrative mechanisms which could undertake, or assist in undertaking the work proposed. *A National Commission of Inquiry* working with the cooperation of the Departments of Education and Science, and Health and Social Security, would have the greatest national legitimacy provided that its membership was truly representative and committed to reaching workable compromises on the more controversial issues. Models for such a commission exist in the form perhaps of the Kingman Commission on the teaching of the English language. Such a commission would be appointed by the Secretary of State with the aim of addressing an agenda in order to provide serious directives relating to the issues listed above. It would also be obliged to arrive at principles governing the subject, as well as methodological guidelines to assist teachers at the classroom level, and bodies such as the school governing board which have been given new responsibilities in this area but as yet little practical assistance. It would draw upon written and oral evidence from the spectrum of educational, medical, moral- religious, academic and other organisational interests. International developments would be invaluable in such an exercise. It would take as its background, the history of state involvement in the subject and the future significance of the national curriculum.

Alternative though perhaps less authoritative mechanisms might include:

- a Department of Education and Science *research project* (or even an independent university-based project);
- a specially-created partnership involving representatives of teachers, head teachers, parents, school governors, local educational authorities, religious bodies etc. to advise the National Curriculum Council.
- creation of *Joint Action Committee* on Sex Education as representative body of spectrum of independent interest groups, which would include the full spectrum of 'political' interests:

including the National Children's Bureau, the Family Planning Association, and other relevant NGOs.

The absence of national guidelines to deal with these factors leaves local initiatives exposed to the continuous threat of 'scandalisation' and other forms of sabotage. Regulation by a nationally recognised authority would offer teachers (observing guidelines) some defence against this. Sex educators need the support of 'official' guidelines which carry an authority which cannot come from methodologies offered within the commercial market, such as the pilloried *Taught not Caught* of the Clarity Collective.(10) As Boëthius has noted, it was the early government guidelines in Sweden which gave teachers the courage to start sex education, as they could rely upon the official support of the Central Board of Schools to which public or media criticism could be deflected, mistakes being corrected by the refinements of successive review commissions (see chapter 6.1). However, securing teacher motivation is only part of the problem. Many brave and enthusiastic efforts have been subverted by the exploitation of school sex education by outside 'political' interests, whether local politicians looking for a means to increase their popularity by scandal-mongering, or journalists seeking sensationalism for profit.(11)

It is difficult to conceive of British school sex education continuing as a covert enterprise of those teachers daring or interested enough to conduct it. Nor in the current political climate has any relevant national organisation the mandate to mediate between traditionalistic and progressive interests, which could be undertaken by a National Commission independent of party political control.

Within both the 'traditionalist' and 'progressive' sex education tendencies, there is a sense that sex education is in part a personal skill which cannot easily be acquired by following rules or training. While this may be true it does not invalidate the creation of an elaborated, regulated field of training which offers teachers, to whom the subject does not come easily, the means to avoid straying beyond boundaries dictated by the limitations of the classroom. Belief in sex education as the vocational preserve of the sexually 'balanced' adult will serve only to mystify the subject and overstate what the school can achieve in the ethics field.

On the contrary, school sex education must evolve into a routine, uncontroversial and 'open' subject with an explicit theory and practice which is seen to acknowledge the moral convictions of the *majority* of the population. It cannot be made the servant of minority interests on the right or left. Rules are required not only to inspire confidence that a correct and endorsed path is being followed, but also as a means to ensure teacher conformity. In this respect, ideally, it should be possible for Christians, Marxists or gays to provide such education according to rules which compartmentalise their personal and 'public' selves etc. If such a compartmentalisation were not acceptable to those espousing such identities, then they would be no more suitable to teach any other school subject in which values arise. Had such guidelines already been in existence, the grotesque *Local Government (Amendment) Bill* forbidding the 'promotion' of homosexuality by local authorities responsible for education would not have been considered.

The impact of AIDS: the threat of AIDS has served to increase the involvement of national government in the design of sex education, though this has been more directed to media advertising than schools as such. This has so far served to cut through much traditionalistic resistance to exposure of contraceptives to all age groups. The long term impact of the AIDS crisis on the core problems of sex education can only be guessed at, though it is already clear that one price to be paid for exposing to the public consciousness otherwise forbidden details of sexual behaviour and contraception will be to force sex education towards the disease-prevention rationale from which so many had fought to rescue it, in pursuit of a more humanistic positive treatment of sexual desire.

Notes

1. Davies, C 'Moralists, Causalists, Sex, Law and Morality' in Armytage, W, Chester, R & Peel, J eds *Changing Patterns of Sexual Behaviour* Academic Press 1980 pg 38

2. Department of Education and Science *Health Education from 5 - 16* Curriculum Matters 6 HMSO 1986

3. Bury, J *Teenage Pregnancy in Britain* Birth Control Trust 1984

4. Doggett, A-M in Allen, E *Education in Sex and Personal Relationships* Policy Studies Institute, London pg 221

5. excluding political parties

6. see for example: White, M and Kidd, J *Sound Sex Education: Preparation for Marriage and Parenthood* Order of Christian Unity. Recommended seven safeguards to prevent unprincipled propaganda from entering the classroom:

- parents rights to know the content of school sex education;
- strengthening head teachers' responsibilities in this area;
- teachers ('ideally a happily married man or woman')(1976:9) to be approved by head teachers and Health Education Authorities;
- teachers to be thoroughly investigated;
- contraceptive education to emphasize failure rates and dangers;
- health hazards of promiscuity to be stressed;

- the use of existing laws to protect children from 'obscene' material.

The Responsible Society has proposed its own albeit dogmatic version (*Sex Education in Schools : What Every parent Should Know* May 1982):

- 'Respect for infant life before and after birth should be an ideal set before children throughout all sex instruction and education.
- Any instruction given to school children on the act of sexual intercourse or human reproduction should be given in the context of marriage.
- Teachers or visiting speakers should not teach, discuss or use printed material which instructs children in unlawful, unnatural, perverse or deviant sexual practices.
- Any act which would constitute an offence against public decency were it to be carried out in public should not be performed, demonstrated or exhibited in pictorial form to or in front of children in schools.
- Coarse, indecent and obscene terminology should be avoided at all time in schools; the language used by all teachers and visiting speakers should be dignified in accordance with the principles and guidelines above.
- Discussion, teaching and/or instruction in the use of contraceptives should be given in the context of marriage and not given to children below the age of consent (16 years). There should be no implication in such instruction, teaching or discussion that it is anticipated that schoolchildren are likely to be involved in any kind of unlawful sexual intercourse.
- Any kind of pornographic or indecent book or other printed text, cinematograph or television films, slides, video-cassettes or other representations should be excluded from all teaching, discussion or instruction in schools.'

In contrast, the following guidelines have been proposed by a working group on the other side of the political spectrum:

'Material brought from a variety of sources should be used to produce material which:

- states that sexual feelings are natural for people regardless of age or sex and such feelings represent a basis for mutual enjoyment;
- examines the nature of male and female sexuality and the resulting attitudes;
- provides honest accurate and straightforward information;

- deals with the emotions and responsibilities of sexuality and discusses alternatives to heterosexuality and marriage. (George Green School Community Education Project, *Who Tells the Children?* Teachers' Notes on Sex Education Manchester 1979)

7. Dallas, D *Sex Education in School and Society* NFER 1972.

8. Doggett in Allen op cit. pg 221.

9. The National Council of Women of Great Britain *Sex Education: Whose Responsibility?* The Council 1984

10. Dixon, H & Mullinar, G (English edition editors) *Taught Not Caught: Strategies for Sex Education* Clarity Collective, Literary Development Aids, Cambridge 1983.

11. see Muraskin L & Jargowsky, P *Creating and Implementing Family Life Education in New Jersey* National Association of State Boards of Education 1985. This study provides an important account of the development of one of the best sex education programmes in any US state; particularly the process of consultation, creation of committees, and securing of political support from a range of otherwise competing interests for the school programme. The programme nevertheless failed to fulfil its original intentions, programmatic goals and rationales were successively diluted in the face of political interference for reasons not always connected with sex education itself:

> 'Political opposition led to a compromise and a major change in the extent to which famiy life education was state defined. Both conservative activists and leaders of most of the state's education associations attacked the proposed requirement. The state's legislature threatened to take action which would stop the policy from being enacted. With continued support from the health and social welfare establishments as well as the backing of the New Jersey Conference of Catholic Bishops, the Board was able to save the overall policy. It was forced, however, to make changes which limited the state's ability to define practice.'... 'The content and nature of instruction.. were left to the local school districts.' (pg 1)

As a result, beyond curriculum development most of the districts did not undertake major implementation efforts.

Appendix

The Origin and Methodology of the Study

The International Planned Parenthood Federation

The IPPF is the world's leading voluntary family planning organisation. It is a federation of autonomous family planning associations in over 120 countries. Founded in 1952, its aims are: to initiate and support family planning services throughout the world, and to increase understanding by people and governments of the interrelated issues of population, resources, environment and development.

Europe is one of the six Regions of the Federation, comprising 22 national FPAs. The IPPF has been concerned for many years with the special needs, desires and problems of adolescents in their sexual development, and with alleviating these problems with appropriate education and health services. Its work is guided by the following Regional Strategies:

-   urging family planning associations to exert pressure on their governments to provide planned parenthood education and services in health, social and educational structures, and for appropriate legal changes;

-   reaffirming the Region's commitment to the fundamental human right of people to determine freely the number and spacing of their children, regardless of demographic considerations;

-   encouraging social reforms which effectively implement the human right to determine freely the number and spacing of children, and the equal rights of both sexes.

A recent IPPF Europe Region investigation of planned parenthood laws, and the services to which they relate, confirmed that a transformation had occurred over two decades in the policies of European governments towards the provision of assistance with contraceptive services (1). It is fair to say that, in the majority of countries in the Region, this applies, to some extent, to young people as well as the adult population. However, for a number of reasons this does not extend to family life and sex education through schools. National laws and regulations, while amenable to the principle of family life/sex education, in few cases extend as far as nationally-endorsed curriculum guidelines which guarantee a minimum standard and 'quantity' of teaching. Even where a nationally-standardised curriculum for family life and sex education has been designed, there remain problems connected with the effective implementation of such curricula and the motivation of teaching staff. While there are many reasons for this state of affairs, some of which are addressed in this study, it is possible to perceive a cross-fertilisation of ideas and systems throughout Europe (the Scandinavian experience having particular influence in Eastern as well as Western Europe), and a common movement toward governmental involvement and standardisation of theory and practice.

This was already identified in an IPPF Europe report of 1975:

> 'It is clear, as we might have guessed, that changes in the legal status of sex education, even the favourable disposition of the Ministry or Department of Education, are not enough to ensure the widespread implementation of sex education in schools. Far more important than this is the approval of teachers and their endorsement of sex education programmes if they are to be implemented on any large scale. We have to recognise that teachers are often defensive, resistant and resentful of changes brought into schools particularly where these changes are legally imposed without teacher participation from the beginning.'(2)

This unsatisfactory relationship between law-maker and teacher is further complicated by the activities of other official and unofficial bureaucracies and pressure groups concerned to influence the teaching of this subject. As well as the problem posed by interpersonal and administrative obstacles to teaching practice, there exists that of creating a suitable knowledge base on which teachers can feel confident to draw, which will not automatically generate criticism or opposition.

As long ago as 1972, the Consultative Assembly of the Council of Europe implied that the creation of 'a common body of information (on sex education) which would be transmitted to pupils at different levels' was a practical possibility for member states. (3)

The Europe Region Project

At the Europe Regional Council 1985, the Regional bureau submitted a project to investigate:

- the relative influence of government and non-governmental (professional) interest groups on the establishment of a national sex education rationale and curricula;
- the political-administrative processes which govern the implementation of sex education curricula in schools;

- the role and status of the FPA, compared with other interest groups (including the government) in contributing to effective teaching practice, and how to improve this status.

In the light of the above, it was proposed that a limited number of European FPA contact persons undertake an investigation of sex/family life education with reference to two dimensions.

1. The Ideological Dimension:

It is intended here to examine the ethical, philosophical and sociological bases on which the most important sex/family life educational policies (rationale, curriculum guidelines and content) are established. This concerns both the interpretation placed on sexuality itself, and the rationale for its delivery as a curriculum item. The FPA is seen as one of several (potential) contributors to this 'formula', which will finally be adopted by (certain) schools.

2. The Social-Structural Dimension:

It is intended here to expose the (hidden) social structure through which the ideological dimension is negotiated, manipulated, implemented. This refers to the 'systems' (bureaucratic, administrative, political) which together make up the social context in which sex education is created. It refers not only to the 'classroom' but the many other important systems or sub-systems (eg. the school governing body, Ministry of Health, FPA etc) which influence, positively or negatively, what teachers offer to their pupils.

Methodology

The Regional Executive Committee requested a 1985 Programme Working Group to suggest a short-list of countries where sex education had developed in contrasting ways, reflecting religious, legal and other cultural differences.

The resulting working group was comprised of the following countries and participants, whose work was coordinated by Dr. Philip Meredith, IPPF:

Belgium: (Flemish-speaking: Dr. Freddy Deven/ Francophone: Mrs. Hélène Aronis-Brykman)

Denmark: (Dr. Hanne Risør)

Federal Republic of Germany: (Mr. Karl-Ernst Plümer)

German Democratic Republic: (Dr. Claus Drunkenmölle)

Poland: (Prof.Mikolaj Kozakiewicz)

Turkey: (Dr. Semra Koral)

United Kingdom: (Mr. Alan Beattie)

It was agreed that this core group would meet bi-annually within a three-year phased project to initiate a 7 country research programme which, in the final year, would be extended to other interested countries.

The 7 country methodology comprises a combination of content analysis of relevant literature, legal decisions, curriculum aids etc., and a selection of interviews of significant individuals (including for example: representatives of: political parties/ government ministries; media; school boards; educational authorities; sex education pedagogues; FPA and other organisations such as the Catholic Church). The group has also attempted to standardise the content of their interviews to cover among other things: history of sex education provision; rationale behind school curriculum; theory or theories of sexuality; management of facts versus values in the curriculum etc.

An IPPF report containing the country studies is forthcoming in 1989.

Notes

1. Meredith, P and Thomas, L eds *Planned Parenthood in Europe* Croom Helm 1986
2. Kozakiewicz, M and Rea, N *A Survey on the Status of Sex Education in European Member Countries* IPPF Europe 1975, pg 68
3. Council of Europe, European Commission of Human Rights: *Case Kjeldsen, Busk Madsen and Pedersen* Report of the Commission, Strasbourg 1975 pg 32

Selected Bibliographical References

Allen, I *Education in Sex and Personal Relationships* Policy Studies Institute 1987.

Archer, J and Lloyd, B *Sex and Gender* Penguin Harmondsworth 1982.

Bernstein, B *Class, Codes and Control* Vol 1, *Theoretical Studies Towards a Sociology of Language*, London, Routledge & Kegan Paul 1977.

Boëthius, C G *Current Sweden* No 315 Svenska Institutet, Box 7434 S-103 91 Stockholm 1984.

Braestrup, A *Sex Education in Denmark* Foreningen for Familieplanlaegning, Copenhagen 1973.

Bury, J *Teenage Pregnancy in Britain* Birth Control Trust 1984

Coote, A and Campbell, B *Sweet Freedom: The Struggle for Women's Liberation* Picador 1982.

Council of Europe: European Commission of Human Rights *Case of Kjeldsen, Busk Madsen and Pedersen* Report of the Commission, Strasbourg 1975; Judgement 1976.

Cousins, J *Make it Happy* Virago 1978.

Dallas, D *Sex Education in School and Society* NFER 1972.

Davies, C 'Moralists, Causalists, Sex, Law and Morality' in Armytage, W, Chester, R and Peel, J eds *Changing Patterns of Sexual Behaviour* Academic Press 1980.

Department of Education and Science *Health Education from 5 - 16* Curriculum Matters 6 HMSO 1986.

Dixon, H and Mullinar, G (English edition editors) *Taught Not Caught: Strategies for Sex Education* Clarity Collective, Literary Development Aids, Cambridge 1983.

Doggett, A-M in Allen, E *Education in Sex and Personal Relationships* Policy Studies Institute, London 1987

Douglas, M *Natural Symbols*, Pelican, Penguin, Harmondsworth 1973.

Farrell, C *My Mother Said...The Way Young People Learned about Sex* Routledge & Kegan Paul 1978.

Gluck, G and Schliewert, H-J *Schule: der richtige Ort für die Sexualerziehung? Ergebnisse einer empirischen Untersuchung* RWTH Aachen, Sem. für Schulpsdagogik und Allgemeine Didaktik, Aachen 1987.

Habermas, J *Knowledge and Human Interests* Heinemann London 1978.

Halmos, P *The Faith of the Counsellors* Constable, London 1965.

Hansen, S and Jensen, J *The Little Red Schoolbook* Stage 1 (English Translation 1971).

Heraud, B J *Sociology and Social Work: Perspectives and Problems* Pergamon Press, Oxford 1970.

Jackson, S *Sexuality and Childhood* Blackwell, Oxford 1982

Kinsey, A *et al. Sexual Behaviour in the Human Male* Saunders, Philadelphia 1948.

Kinsey, A *et al. Sexual Behaviour in the Human Female* Saunders, Philadelphia 1953.

Kozakiewicz, M, 'The History and Politics of Planned Parenthood Laws in Poland' in Meredith, P & Thomas, L eds *Planned Parenthood in Europe* Croom Helm, London 1986.

Kozakiewicz, M and Rea, N *Sex Education and Adolescence in Europe* IPPF Europe London 1975.

Lee, Carol *The Ostrich Position* Readers and Writers, London 1983.

Leth, I, Skalts, V and Hoffmeyer, E *Sex Education in Primary and Secondary Schools in Denmark* 1961 (English summary).

Lukes, S *Power: A Radical View*, Blackwell, London, 1975.

Meredith, P and Thomas, L eds. *Planned Parenthood in Europe* Croom Helm, London 1986.

Meredith, P ed. *The Other Curriculum: European Strategies for School Sex Education* IPPF Europe 1989 .

Mitchell, J *Psychoanalysis and Feminism* Allen Lane, London 1974.

Myrdal, A and G *Crisis and Population* 1934 (English version: Myrdal, *A Nation and Family* 1941) MIT Press (Cambridge 1968).

The National Council of Women of Great Britain *Sex Education: Whose Responsibility?* The Council 1984.

National Swedish Board of Education *Instruction Concerning Interpersonal Relations* Liber Utbildningsforlaget Stockholm 1981.

Newsom, J *The Education of Girls* Faber & Faber 1948.

Plummer, K *Sexual Stigma: An Interactionist Account* Routledge & Kegan Paul London 1975.

Population Crisis Committee *World Access to Birth Control* Washington DC 1987.

RFSU *Vision, Reality, Activities* PO Box 17006, S-104 62 Stockholm 1981

Reiff, P *The Triumph of the Therapeutic* Penguin, Harmondsworth 1966

Reiss, I L *Journey Into Sexuality* Prentice-Hall, Englewood Cliffs, New Jersey 1986.

Robinson, P A *The Sexual Radicals: Reich, Roheim, Marcuse* Paladin, London 1972.

Schofield, M *The Sexual Behaviour of Young People* Longman London 1965

Schofield, M *The Sexual Behaviour of Young Adults* Allen Lane, London 1973

Skaumal, U *Richlinien zur Sexualerziehung* IPN-Materialen, Kiel 1986

Swedish National Board of Education *Instruction Concerning Interpersonal Relations* 1981 Liber Stockholm 1981

Szasz, T 'The Case against Sex Education' *British Journal of Medicine* Vol 8 December 1981.

United Nations: *Report of the International Conference on Population* Mexico City 6-14 August 1984 UN New York 1984 (E/conf 76/19).

Wallis, Geoffrey. P *Some Ideological Issues in Sex Education in Post-War Britain* unpublished MA Dissertation. University of London Institute of Education September 1984.

Wallis, G 1984 op cit. pg 92, quoting McIntosh, M in Women's Study Group (eds) *Women Take Issue*: Aspects of Women's Subordination Centre for Contemporary Cultural Studies, Hutchinson Birmingham 1978.

Weeks, J *Sex, Politics and Society: The Regulation of Sexuality Since 1800* Longman, Harlow 1981.

Weeks, J *Sexuality and Its Discontents: Meanings, Myths and Modern Sexualities* Routledge & Kegan Paul, London 1985.

Weeks, J *Sexuality* Ellis Horwood/ Tavistock Publications, London 1986.

Weeks, J *Sexuality* Tavistock 1986.

Index

Society for Conscious Motherhood 150
sociobiology 48
sociology 51
Solidarity 153
Soviet Union 151
Swedish Family Planning Association 101
Swedish National Board of Education 102
Swinton, Earl of 28
Szasz, Thomas 3, 4

T

teenage pregnancy 119
therapy 47
Third Reich 136
traditionalists 20

U

United Nations 3
USA 2, 4

V

value-neutrality 105

W

Wallis, G 46
Weeks, Jeffrey 43, 63
Widerström, K 101

Z

Zetterberg, H 104